Name of Institution...................................................................

# CERTIFICATE

This is to certify that
Mr./Miss...................................
Roll No...................has satisfactorily completed
the exercises in Oral Pathology & Microbiology
as prescribed by the Department of Oral Pathology
& Microbiology for B.D.S. 3rd Year Course, in the
laboratory of this Institution in the academic year
..........................

Date....................... Teacher-in-charge.......................

Head of the Department.............................

Date of Practical Examination: ................................................

Signature of Examiners: 1)......................... 2)..........................

# Manual of Oral Pathology

## For the Students of Dentistry

*(A Manual to be Used for the Practical Classes in Oral Pathology and Microbiology)*

**Dr. Susmita Saxena,** MDS
Prof. and Head
Department of Oral Pathology
ESIC Dental College & Hospital
Rohini, New Delhi

**SECOND EDITION**

*To Access Images go to link*
**goo.gl/oqHqjc**

**PEEPEE**
**PUBLISHERS AND DISTRIBUTORS (P) LTD.**

**Manual of Oral Pathology**

*Published by:*
**Pawaninder P. Vij**
Peepee Publishers and Distributors (P) Ltd.
*Head Office:* 160, Shakti Vihar, Pitam Pura
New Delhi-110 034

***Correspondence Address:***

**7/31, Ansari Road, Daryaganj**
**New Delhi-110002 (India)**

**Ph: 41512412, 23246245, 9811156083**

***e-mail:* peepee160@yahoo.co.in**

***e-mail:* peepee160@gmail.com**

**www.peepeepub.com**



*First Edition:* 2006
**Second Edition: 2017, 2019, 2022, 2023**

**ISBN:** 9788184452280

# Preface to the Second Edition

This Oral Pathology Manual was designed to guide the undergraduate students in essential aspects of Oral Pathology through histopathology slides and specimens. Abridged theory provided with each topic will enable students to experience and prepare for commonly asked viva-voce questions. It was necessary to add a chapter on Forensic Odontology as it has been recently included in the BDS syllabus and students need to be aware of this branch of dentistry when they become graduates. Some relevant simple exercises can be undertaken in Practical classes which will make the students interested in this fairly new subject. Rest of the topics remain the same as in the previous edition of the Manual, thus sufficing the training as required in undergraduate classes of BDS. I sincere wish that students will at least read through the text of this manual before appearing for viva and practical exams when there is insufficient time to revise the complete syllabus.

***Susmita Saxena***

# Preface to the First Edition

While teaching the undergraduate students of BDS for the past fifteen years, I realized that there was a lack of structured training in Oral Pathology as far as the practical classes are concerned. This manual has been designed solely for the purpose of laboratory/practical classes where specimens, models and histopathologic slides are shown so that the student is well versed with the basic requirement of the subject before appearing for the Practical examination in Oral Pathology and Microbiology. Topics where slides or specimens are not normally shown have been covered in a questionnaire form which may be completed by the students in the class which will improve their theoretical knowledge as well. Brief descriptions of the topics have been included in this manual based on the standard textbooks of "A Textbook of Oral Pathology" by Shafer, Hine and Levy—4th Edition and "Oral and Maxillofacial Pathology" by Neville, Damm, Allen and Bouquot—2nd Edition. Only the "must know" topics of Oral Pathology have been included for the undergraduate students of Dentistry which most examiners would expect the students to be aware of, along with a CD of commonly shown specimens and slides.

***Susmita Saxena***

# Acknowledgements

A sincere thanks goes out to all my undergraduate students who read, understood and performed well in their exams. I wish to thank all the teachers of Oral Pathology who are following this Manual and have found it useful in training their students. It gives me great satisfaction to see that the practical exercises in Oral Pathology have become more structured and systematic by following this Manual.

Once again my thanks to Mr. Pawaninder Pal Vij of Peepee publishers and Distributors for reminding me of the need for a second edition of the Manual.

***Susmita Saxena***

# Contents



*To Access*
*Images go to link*
**goo.gl/oqHqjc**

# INDEX

| Sl No | Topic | Page No | Grade | Signature |
|---|---|---|---|---|
| | | | | |
| | | | | |
| | | | | |
| | | | | |
| | | | | |
| | | | | |
| | | | | |
| | | | | |
| | | | | |
| | | | | |
| | | | | |
| | | | | |
| | | | | |
| | | | | |
| | | | | |
| | | | | |
| | | | | |
| | | | | |
| | | | | |
| | | | | |
| | | | | |
| | | | | |
| | | | | |
| | | | | |
| | | | | |
| | | | | |
| | | | | |
| | | | | |

# INDEX

| Sl No | Topic | Page No | Grade | Signature |
|---|---|---|---|---|
| | | | | |
| | | | | |
| | | | | |
| | | | | |
| | | | | |
| | | | | |
| | | | | |
| | | | | |
| | | | | |
| | | | | |
| | | | | |
| | | | | |
| | | | | |
| | | | | |
| | | | | |
| | | | | |
| | | | | |
| | | | | |
| | | | | |
| | | | | |
| | | | | |
| | | | | |
| | | | | |
| | | | | |
| | | | | |
| | | | | |
| | | | | |
| | | | | |

# INDEX

| Sl No | Topic | Page No | Grade | Signature |
|---|---|---|---|---|
| | | | | |
| | | | | |
| | | | | |
| | | | | |
| | | | | |
| | | | | |
| | | | | |
| | | | | |
| | | | | |
| | | | | |
| | | | | |
| | | | | |
| | | | | |
| | | | | |
| | | | | |
| | | | | |
| | | | | |
| | | | | |
| | | | | |
| | | | | |
| | | | | |
| | | | | |
| | | | | |
| | | | | |
| | | | | |
| | | | | |
| | | | | |
| | | | | |

# INDEX

| Sl No | Topic | Page No | Grade | Signature |
|---|---|---|---|---|
| | | | | |
| | | | | |
| | | | | |
| | | | | |
| | | | | |
| | | | | |
| | | | | |
| | | | | |
| | | | | |
| | | | | |
| | | | | |
| | | | | |
| | | | | |
| | | | | |
| | | | | |
| | | | | |
| | | | | |
| | | | | |
| | | | | |
| | | | | |
| | | | | |
| | | | | |
| | | | | |
| | | | | |
| | | | | |
| | | | | |
| | | | | |
| | | | | |

Exercise One

# DEVELOPMENTAL DISORDERS OF ORAL STRUCTURES

**CONGENITAL DISEASE:** A disease, which is present at or before birth but is not necessarily, inherited i.e. transmitted through the genes.

**HEREDITARY DISEASE:** Conditions, which are apparent at birth or may manifest over a number of years after birth and are transmitted through the genes.

## CAUSES OF CONGENITAL DEVELOPMENTAL ANOMALIES

A. Genetic factors:
1. Inherited
2. Mutagenetic

B. Environmental factors:
1. Infections
2. Physical injuries
3. Hormonal influence
4. Nutritional abnormalities
5. Respiration
6. Drugs and chemicals
7. Maternal diseases and defects
8. Embryonic defects.

## SPECIMENS SHOWING DEVELOPMENTAL DISORDERS OF TEETH

1. **Gemination:** An attempt at division of a single tooth germ by an invagination, with resultant incomplete formation of two teeth. A tooth with two completely or incompletely separated crowns with a single root or root canal.

**2. Fusion:** Union of two normally separated tooth germs gives rise to fused teeth, which may be complete or incomplete. The tooth may have separate or fused root canals.

3. **Concrescence:** Concrescence is fusion of teeth occurring after the completion of root formation. The teeth are joined together by deposition of cementum.

4. **Dilaceration:** An abnormal angulation or bend in the root or, less frequently, the crown of a tooth is called dilaceration.

5. **Talon cusp:** A talon cusp is a well-delineated additional cusp resembling an eagle's talon that is located lingually from cingulum area extending to the incisal edge of maxillary or mandibular permanent incisors.

6. **Dens invaginatus:** "Dens in dente" is a developmental variation, which is thought to arise as a result of an invagination in the surface of a tooth crown before calcification has occurred. May be of coronal type or radicular type.

**7. Dens evaginatus:** Dens evaginatus is a cusplike globule of enamel located on the occlusal surface between the buccal and lingual cusps of premolars and rarely on molars.

**8. Taurodontism:** Taurodontism is a dental anomaly in which the body of the tooth is enlarged at the expense of the roots. These teeth resemble the teeth of cud-chewing animals and may be further classified into hypotaurodont, mesotaurodont and hypertaurodont depending upon the degree of apical displacement of the pulpal floor.

9. **Supernumerary roots:** The term supernumerary roots refers to the development of an increased number of roots on a tooth compared with that classically described in dental anatomy.

## DEVELOPMENTAL DISORDERS AFFECTING NUMBER OF TEETH

**Anodontia:** Define Anodontia. Name a condition showing generalized anodontia.

**Supernumerary teeth:** Which teeth commonly occur as supernumerary teeth. Name some syndromes associated with supernumerary teeth.

Define the following:

*Predeciduous dentition.*

*Natal teeth.*

*Neonatal teeth.*

*Postpermanent dentition.*

## DEVELOPMENTAL DISORDERS AFFECTING STRUCTURE OF TEETH

Amelogenesis imperfecta—also known as:
Types of amelogenesis imperfecta:

Name the environmental causes of enamel hypoplasia.

Describe mottled enamel.

What is Turner's hypoplasia?

Classify dentinogenesis imperfecta. Write the features of each type.

Describe rootless teeth.

What are 'Ghost teeth'? Give the synonyms for ghost teeth.

## DEVELOPMENTAL DISTURBANCES AFFECTING THE JAWS

Name the developmental disorders of the jaws.

**Describe Parry:** Romberg syndrome.

## DEVELOPMENTAL DISTURBANCES AFFECTING LIPS AND PALATE

Draw and label the processes forming the face.

Non-fusion of which processes gives rise to the following conditions:

1. **Commissural pits and fistulas.**

2. **Cleft lip.**

3. **Cleft palate.**

Describe the following:

1. **Cheilitis glandularis.**

2. **Cheilitis granulomatosa.**

3. **Peutz-Jeghers syndrome.**

## DEVELOPMENTAL DISTURBANCES AFFECTING ORAL MUCOSA AND GINGIVA

1. Fordyce's granules.

2. Focal epithelial hyperplasia.

3. Fibromatosis gingiva.

## DEVELOPMENTAL DISTURBANCES AFFECTING THE TONGUE

1. **Aglossia:** Describe the development of tongue.

2. **Microglossia.**

3. **Macroglossia.**

4. **Ankyloglossia:** What is "tongue-tie"? What causes ankyloglossia?

5. **Cleft tongue:** Non-fusion of which processes causes cleft tongue?

6. **Fissured tongue:** What is the other name for it? Draw the different types on the basis of clinical appearance.

7. **Median rhomboid glossitis:** How does it arise? What may be the causative organism?

8. **Benign migratory glossitis:** What are the other names? Describe clinical appearance. Draw the histologic picture.

9. **Hairy tongue:** What are the possible causative factors? Usually associated with which infection?

10. **Lingual varices:** Which veins of the tongue normally show varices?

11. **Lingual thyroid nodule:** Describe the development of thyroid gland.

## DEVELOPMENTAL DISTURBANCES AFFECTING SALIVARY GLANDS

1. **Aplasia:** Describe the development of salivary gland. Enumerate the causes of xerostomia.

2. **Developmental lingual mandibular salivary gland depression:** What is the other name? Describe why it occurs.

**Exercise Two**

# REGRESSIVE ALTERATIONS OF THE TEETH

Tooth structure can be lost after its formation by a variety of influences beyond the obvious cases related to caries or traumatic fractures. Destruction can begin on the enamel surface of the crown through abrasion, attrition, erosion or abfraction. In addition, loss of tooth structure can begin on the dentin or cemented surfaces of the teeth by external or internal resorption.

1. What is the physiologic wearing away of tooth structure called?

2. Identify the specimens showing attrition, abrasion, and erosion and describe their clinical features.

3. Abfraction (stress-induced cervical lesions).

Abfraction means, "to break away" and is a term used in dentistry to define the pathologic loss of tooth structure at, or under, the cemento-enamel junction caused by abnormal biomechanical loading. Abfraction appears as a sharp, wedge-shaped, or V-shaped defect of enamel and dentin along the cervical region of the facial aspect of a tooth.

4. **Internal and External resorption:** In addition to loss of tooth structure that begins on the exposed coronal surfaces, destruction of teeth also can occur through resorption, which is accomplished by cells located in the dental pulp (i.e. internal resorption) or in the periodontal ligament (i.e. external resorption).
What are the causes of Internal resorption?

Enumerate the factors associated with External resorption.

**Regressive changes of the pulp**

1. Reticular atrophy.
2. Pulp calcification:
   a. True denticles
   b. False denticles
   c. Diffuse calcification

**Hypercementosis**

A regressive change of teeth characterized by the deposition of excessive amounts of secondary cementum on root surfaces.

## DISCOLORATION OF TEETH

Abnormal colorations may be extrinsic (i.e., arising from the surface accumulation of exogenous pigment) or intrinsic (i.e., secondary to endogenous factors that result in the discoloration of the underlying dentin).

Enumerate the causes of extrinsic staining of teeth.

Enumerate the causes of intrinsic staining of teeth.

Exercise Three

# BENIGN AND MALIGNANT TUMOURS OF THE ORAL CAVITY

The word "tumour" means a swelling of the tissue.
A neoplasm is often considered an independent, uncoordinated new growth of tissue which is potentially capable of unlimited proliferation and which does not regress after removal of the stimulus, which produced the lesion.

## TUMOURS OF EPITHELIAL TISSUE ORIGIN

**BENIGN:**
1. **Papilloma:** The papilloma is an exophytic proliferation of stratified squamous epithelium resulting in a papillary or verruciform mass.
***Histopathologic Features:*** The papilloma is characterized by a proliferation of keratinized stratified squamous epithelium arrayed in fingerlike projections with fibrovascular connective tissue cores.

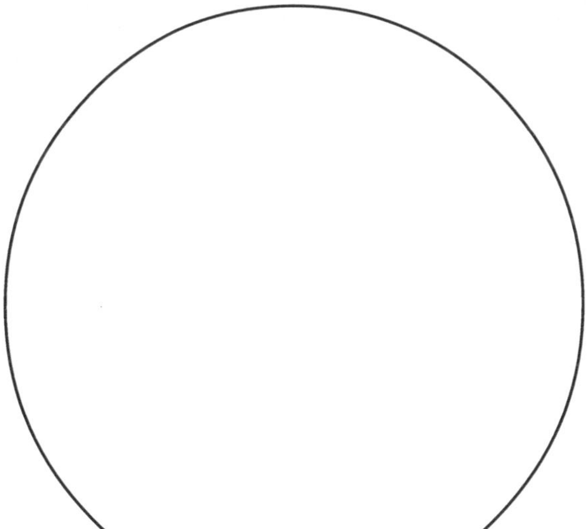

2. **Keratoacanthoma:** It is also known as self-healing carcinoma. This benign epithelial lesion resembles epidermoid carcinoma clinically and histologically.
Describe the clinical course of keratoacanthoma.

***Histopathologic Features:*** It consists of hyperparakeratinized hyperplastic stratified squamous epithelium with keratin plugging. The margin of the lesion is characteristic where adjacent normal epithelium is elevated toward the central portion of the crater and forms an acute angle with the lesion.

3. **Pigmented cellular nevus:** A nevus is a congenital, developmental tumour-like malformation of the skin or mucous membrane. The pigmented nevus is a superficial lesion composed of "nevus cells" which are derived from neural crest.

What are the types of developmental nevus and acquired nevus?

***Histopathologic Features:*** The lesion is characterized by a benign, unencapsulated proliferation of small, ovoid cells, which are the nevus cells. These cells tend to be arranged in an alveolar pattern called theques.

## PREMALIGNANT LESIONS AND CONDITIONS

**Premalignant lesion:** A benign, morphologically altered tissue that has a greater than normal risk of malignant transformation.

**Premalignant condition:** A disease or patient habit that does not necessarily alter the clinical appearance of local tissue but is associated with a greater than normal risk of precancerous lesion or cancer development in that tissue. Name some premalignant lesions and premalignant conditions.

**Leukoplakia:** Oral leukoplakia is defined by the World Health Organisation (WHO) as "a white patch or plaque that cannot be characterized clinically or pathologically as any other disease".

What are the etiologic factors of leukoplakia?

Clinically leukoplakia may be of the following types:

1. Mild or thin leukoplakia
2. Homogeneous or thick leukoplakia
3. Granular or Nodular leukoplakia
4. Verrucous leukoplakia
5. Proliferative verrucous leukoplakia

The oral mucous membrane may show scattered patches of redness called Erythroplakia. The intermixed red and white lesion is called Erythroleukoplakia or speckled leukoplakia, which frequently reveals advanced dysplasia upon biopsy.

***Histopathologic Features:*** Microscopically leukoplakia is characterized by hyperorthokeratosis or hyperparakeratosis with or without acanthosis. Dysplastic features may be present ranging from mild, moderate to severe degree as in carcinoma-in-situ.

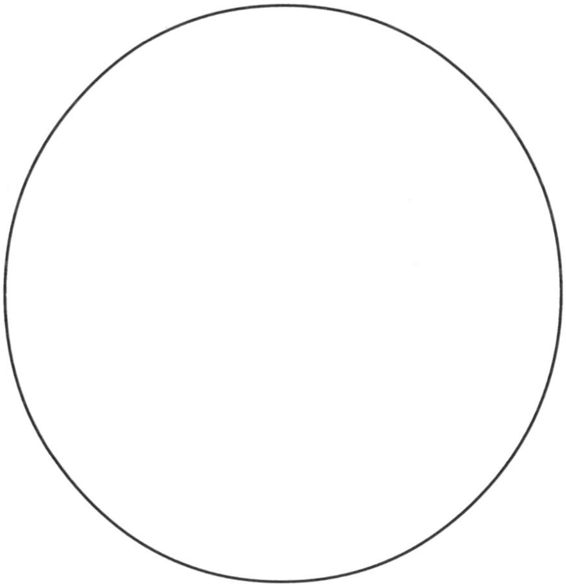

**Erythroplakia:** Erythroplakia is defined as a red patch that cannot be clinically or pathologically diagnosed as any other condition. The etiology of erythroplakia is unknown but presumed to be the same as associated with invasive squamous cell carcinoma of the mouth. Most erythroplakias demonstrate significant epithelial dysplasia, carcinoma-in-situ, or frank invasive carcinoma.

**Intraepithelial carcinoma (Carcinoma-in-situ):** Intraepithelial carcinoma arises frequently on the skin but may also occur in the oral cavity. The clinical appearance may be that of leukoplakia, erythroplakia, speckled leukoplakia, or an ulcerated lesion.

***Histopathologic Features:*** Carcinoma-in-situ is defined as dysplastic epithelial cells that extend from the basal-layer to the surface of the mucosa (top-to-bottom change). Keratin may or may not be present, epithelium may be hyperplastic or atrophic and basement membrane is intact hence metastasis is not seen.

**Oral submucous fibrosis:** Oral submucous fibrosis is a premalignant condition occurring chiefly in Southeast Asia. It is a chronic, progressive, scarring, high-risk condition closely linked with the use of betel quid, which consists of areca nut and slaked lime. The patients develop stiffening of certain areas of the oral mucosa with difficulty in opening the mouth and swallowing.

***Histopathologic Features:*** It is always associated with a juxta-epithelial inflammatory reaction followed by a fibroelastic change of the lamina propria with epithelial atrophy.

Persons with oral submucous fibrosis are at least 19 times more likely to develop oral cancer than persons without the disease.

## MALIGNANT EPITHELIAL TUMOURS

**Basal cell carcinoma:** Basal cell carcinoma is a locally invasive, slowly spreading primary epithelial malignancy that arises from the basal cell layer of the skin and its appendages. This cancer results from chronic exposure to ultraviolet radiation. Oral lesions are seen when there is invasion and infiltration from a skin surface basal cell carcinoma. It is also called Rodent ulcer.

***Histopathologic Features:*** Basal cell carcinoma displays sheets and islands of epithelial cells resembling basal cell layer of skin. Since the basal cell is a pluripotential cell, basal cell carcinoma shows variable microscopic appearances like: Nodulocystic, Superficial, Adenoid, Pigmented, Infiltrative and Keratotic.

**Squamous cell carcinoma:** The epidermoid carcinoma is the most common malignant neoplasm of the oral cavity. The cause of oral squamous cell carcinoma is multifactorial. Extrinsic factors include tobacco smoke, alcohol, syphilis, chronic irritation, viruses and sunlight. Intrinsic factors include systemic or generalized states, such as general malnutrition or iron-deficiency anaemia. Many cases may be associated or preceded by a precancerous lesion, especially leukoplakia. Clinical presentation may be variable, including: Exophytic, Endophytic, Leukoplakic, Erythroplakic or Erythroleukoplakic.

***Histopathologic Features:*** Squamous cell carcinoma arises from dysplastic surface epithelium and is histopathologically characterized by invasive cords and nests of epithelial cells showing malignant changes. Histologic grading of the tumour is done on the basis of degree of resemblance of tumour cells to the parent tissue (squamous epithelium) and production of their normal product keratin. Tumours may be graded as well differentiated, moderately-differentiated or poorly differentiated which predicts prognosis to some extent.

**Staging:** Clinical staging of the tumour is done by tumour-node-metastasis system (TNM) classification, where

T = size of the primary tumour
N = involvement of local lymph nodes
M = distant metastasis.

**Verrucous carcinoma:** Verrucous carcinoma is a low-grade variant of epidermoid carcinoma. This lesion is commonly associated with chronic tobacco or snuff chewing habits and arises typically in the area where the tobacco is habitually placed. Oral lesions appear as exophytic or well-demarcated thick plaques with papillary or verruciform surface projections often covered by a white leukoplakic film.

***Histopathologic Features:*** Lesion shows marked down growth of proliferating epithelium into the connective tissue with wide and elongated rete ridges. Abundant parakeratin is produced with parakeratin plugging in the clefts between the surface projections. The epithelium is well differentiated with significant chronic inflammatory cell infiltration in the underlying connective tissue.

**Malignant melanoma:** Melanoma is a malignant lesion of melanocytic origin, which may arise from a pre-existing benign melanocytic lesion or as a malignant lesion originating from otherwise normal skin or mucosa. There are four clinicopathologic types of melanoma:

1. Superficial-spreading melanoma
2. Nodular melanoma
3. Lentigo maligna melanoma
4. Acral lentiginous melanoma.

Mclanomas exhibit two directional patterns of growth: (1) The radial growth phase, and (2) The vertical growth phase.

***Histopathologic Features:*** Atypical melanocytes are initially seen at the epithelial and connective tissue junction from where they have the potential to proliferate either laterally along the epithelium or downward into the connective tissue. The atypical melanocytes are usually larger than normal melanocytes and have varying degrees of nuclear pleomorphism and hyperchromatism.

## TUMOURS OF CONNECTIVE TISSUE ORIGIN

### BENIGN:

1. **Fibroma:** It is a common benign soft tissue neoplasm of connective tissue origin. It appears as an elevated lesion of normal colour with a smooth surface and a sessile or pedunculated base.

***Histopathologic Features:*** It consists of interlacing bundles of collagenous fibers with varying numbers of fibroblasts and fibrocytes and small blood vessels. The covering stratified squamous epithelium is often atrophic with loss of rete pegs. The microscopic appearance of fibroma is similar to that of an inflammatory hyperplastic lesion. Lesions of the oral cavity are more likely to be focal hyperplasias due to chronic irritation.

2. **Peripheral ossifying fibroma:** It appears clinically as a well-circumscribed focal mass of tissue on the gingiva, which may be sessile or pedunculated or sessile of normal colour or slightly red.

***Histopathologic Features:*** The microscopic appearance of this lesion is that of a fibrous proliferation with a surface stratified squamous epithelium, which may be ulcerated and often covered by a fibrinopurulent membrane with a subjacent zone of granulation tissue. The deeper fibroblastic component is cellular with areas of mineralization. The type of mineralized component is variable and may consist of bone, cementum-like material, or dystrophic calcifications.

3. **Central ossifying fibroma:** This central lesion of bone is similar to central cementifying fibroma, which is an odontogenic tumour. Both these lesions are considered to be fibro-osseous in nature.

***Histopathologic Features:*** The lesion is composed of many delicate interlacing collagen fibers interspersed by large numbers of active proliferating fibroblasts. Presence of characteristic small foci of irregular bony trabeculae, which resembles the bizarre Chinese character of bony trabeculae seen in fibrous dysplasia of bone.

4. **Peripheral giant cell granuloma:** The peripheral giant cell granuloma always occurs on the gingiva or alveolar process as a pedunculated or sessile growth that appears to arise from deeper tissues like either periodontal ligament or mucoperiosteum.

***Histopathologic Features:*** Microscopic examination of this lesion reveals proliferation of multinucleated giant cells within a background of plump ovoid and spindle-shaped fibroblasts and connective tissue fibres. Areas of haemorrhage and inflammatory cell infiltration are also seen.

5. **Central giant cell granuloma:** The central giant cell granuloma is predominantly seen in children or young adults commonly in females and in the mandible. It is characterized by gradual expansion of the jaw and otherwise asymptomatic. X-ray reveals radiolucent area with faint trabeculae and displacement of regional teeth.

***Histopathologic Features:*** The lesion is composed of loose fibrillar connective tissue stroma with proliferating fibroblasts and small capillaries. Multinucleated giant cells are prominent throughout the lesion with areas of extravasated blood and haemosiderin pigment. Osteoid tissue is seen around the periphery of the lesion.

6. **Lipoma:** The lipoma is a benign tumour of fat. Lipomas of the oral and maxillofacial region are much less frequent. Oral lipomas are usually soft, smooth-surfaced nodular masses, which may be sessile or pedunculated with a yellowish hue and a cyst-like feel on palpation.

***Histopathologic Features:*** This well-circumscribed tumour is composed of mature fat cells. Collagen strands course through the lesion with a distinct lobular arrangement of fat cells.

7. **Haemangioma:** The haemangioma is a common tumour of infancy characterized by the proliferation of blood vessels. It is considered to be a hamartoma or a developmental anomaly. It appears as a flat or raised lesion of the mucosa, usually red or bluish-red and seldom well circumscribed.

***Histopathologic Features:*** Numerous plump endothelial cells and vascular spaces containing blood characterize histopathologic features of haemangiomas. Small proliferating vascular channels constitute capillary haemangioma while large blood-filled spaces are characteristic of cavernous haemangiomas.

8. **Lymphangioma:** It is a benign tumour of lymphatic vessels commonly affecting the tongue. The superficial lesions appear papillary while deeper lesions are diffuse nodules or masses.
***Histopathologic Features:*** The cavernous type of lymphangioma is more common which is composed of numerous dilated lymphatics lined by endothelial cells and containing lymph.

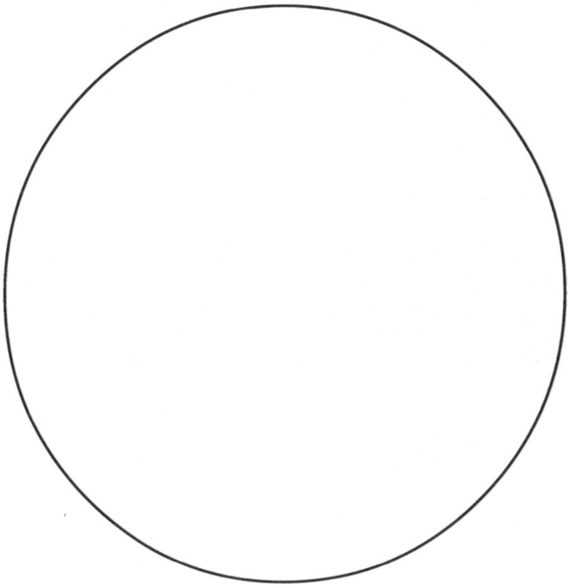

9. **Chondroma:** The chondroma is a benign central tumour of mature cartilaginous tissue, which is uncommon in head and neck region. It arises as a painless slowly progressive swelling of the jaw causing loosening of the teeth. The roentgenogram shows an irregular radiolucent or mottled area in the bone causing root resorption of adjacent teeth.
***Histopathologic Features:*** The chondroma is made up of a mass of hyaline cartilage with uniform small cartilage cells exhibiting areas of calcification or necrosis.

10. **Osteoma:** It is a benign neoplasm of bone, which may arise in an endosteal or periosteal location. Occurrence of oral lesion is uncommon and when it occurs it presents as a circumscribed swelling of the jaw, which is slow growing. X-ray shows a well-circumscribed radiopaque mass within the jaw. The periosteal form of the disease is manifested as a sclerotic mass.

***Histopathologic Features:*** The osteoma is composed of either extremely dense, compact bone or of course cancellous bone. Foci of cartilage may at times be present.

11. **Torus:** Tori are bony protuberance or excrescence of the hard palate or of the mandible. Both torus palatinus and torus mandibularis are hereditary conditions.

***Histopathologic Features:*** The torus palatinus manifests clinically as an outgrowth in the midline of the palate and the overlying mucosa often appears blanched.

The torus mandibularis is an exostosis of bone found on the lingual surface of the mandible usually above the mylohyoid line and opposite the bicuspid teeth.

12. **Traumatic neuroma:** The traumatic neuroma is not a true neoplasm but a reactive proliferation of neural tissue after transection or other damage of a nerve bundle. Repair of the damaged nerve usually occurs unless the proliferating proximal end meets some obstruction, such as scar tissue or a malaligned bone, in which case the nerve continues to proliferate into an unorganized bulbous or nodular mass of nerve fibers and Schwann cells in varying proportions. This constitutes a traumatic neuroma. The oral traumatic neuroma usually appears as a small nodule which is smooth-surfaced and nonulcerated usually occurring in the mental foramen region, tongue and lower lip. A history of trauma often can be elicited.

***Histopathologic Features:*** This lesion characteristically shows a mass of irregular and often interlacing neurofibrils and Schwann cells situated in a scanty or large amount of connective tissue stroma.

13. **Neurofibroma:** The neurofibroma is the most common type of peripheral nerve neoplasm. It arises from Schwann cells, fibroblasts and occasional perineural cells with inermingled neuritis or axons. Neurofibromas can arise as solitary tumours or be a component of neurofibromatosis. They present as slow-growing, painless lesions that vary in size from small nodules to large growths. The tongue and buccal mucosa are the most common intraoral sites.

***Histopathologic Features:*** It is generally composed of a proliferation of delicate spindle cells with thin, wavy nuclei intermingled with neuritis in an irregular pattern as well as delicate, intertwining connective tissue fibrils.

14. **Neurilemoma (Schwannoma):** The neurilemoma is a relatively uncommon, slow-growing, benign neural neoplasm of Schwann cell origin. This encapsulated tumour typically arises in association with a nerve trunk and as it grows it pushes the nerve aside. The tongue is the most common location for intraoral neurilemomas. Intraosseous lesions appear as either unilocular or multilocular radiolucencies on radiographs.

***Histopathologic Features:*** The neurilemoma classically composed of two types of tissue Antoni type A and Antoni type B. Antoni A tissue is characterized by streaming fascicles of spindle-shaped Schwann cells. These cells often form a palisaded arrangement around central acellular eosinophilic areas known as Verocay bodies. Antoni B tissue is less cellular and less organized; the spindle cells are randomly arranged within a loose, myxomatous tissue.

**MALIGNANT:**

1. **Fibrosarcoma:** The fibrosarcoma is a malignant tumour of fibroblasts and may occur in any part of the body where the parent tissue is found. It is relatively uncommon in the head and neck region. They present as slow-growing masses that may reach considerable size before they produce pain.

***Histopathologic Features:*** The fibrosarcoma is characterized by the proliferation of fibroblasts and the formation of collagen and reticulin fibers. Well-differentiated tumours consist of fascicles of spindle-shaped cells that classically form a "herring-bone" pattern. In poorly differentiated tumours, the cells are less organized and show pleomorphism with frequent mitotic activity and tend to produce less collagen.

2. **Liposarcoma:** Liposarcoma is an uncommon malignant mesenchymal neoplasm, especially of the head and neck region. It typically presents as soft, slow-growing painless mass either submucosal or deep in location.

***Histopathologic Features:*** There are five histologic categories of liposarcoma:

(a) Myxoid (b) Round cell (c) Well-differentiated (d) Dedifferentiated (e) Pleomorphic.

The most common of these is the myxoid liposarcoma, which demonstrates proliferating lipoblasts within a myxoid stroma that contains a rich capillary network.

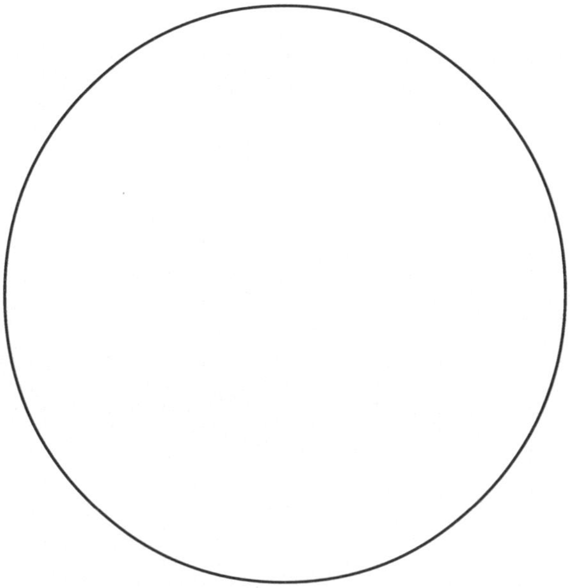

3. **Angiosarcoma:** Angiosarcoma is a rare malignancy of vascular endothelium, which may arise from either blood or lymphatic vessels. More than 50% of all cases occur in the head and neck region, with the scalp and forehead being the most common sites. Oral lesions are quite rare. Cutaneous angiosarcomas of the head and neck are common in elderly and resemble a simple bruise in the early stages, which gradually becomes elevated, nodular with ulcerated surface.

***Histopathologic Features:*** It is characterized by an infiltrative proliferation of endothelium-lined blood vessels that form an anastomosing network. The endothelial cells appear hyperchromatic and atypical and often appear piled up within the vascular lumina.

4. **Kaposi's sarcoma:** Kaposi's sarcoma is an unusual vascular neoplasm that occasionally manifests in the oral cavity. It commonly occurs in individuals infected by (HIV) virus. They appear as reddish or brownish-red nodules of variable sizes and are usually tender or painful. Cervical lymph node and salivary gland involvement is common.
***Histopathologic Features:*** Kaposi's sarcoma typically evolves through three stages: (i) Patch, (ii) Plaque, (iii) Nodular. The lesion is composed of proliferating miniature vessels, which results in an irregular, jagged vascular network that surrounds preexisting vessels. Numerous extravasated erythrocytes are present and slit-like vascular spaces may be discerned.

5. **Chondrosarcoma:** The chondrosarcoma is a malignant tumour of cartilage cells and may occur in either the maxilla or mandible. It may be primary i.e. de novo in origin or may be secondary which arises in a pre-existing chondroma. This tumour manifests as a painless mass or swelling which may be associated with separation or loosening of teeth. Radiographically the tumour presents as a radiolucent lesion with poorly defined borders often containing scattered and variable amounts of radiopaque foci.
***Histopathologic Features:*** The neoplasm is composed of hyaline cartilage with areas of ossification with chondrocytes showing considerable variation in size and shape and binucleated cells are common.

6. **Osteogenic sarcoma:** Osteosarcoma is a malignancy of mesenchymal cells that have the ability to produce osteoid or immature bone. The majority of osteosarcomas demonstrate intramedullary origin, but a small number may be juxtacortical or rarely extraskeletal. Pain and swelling of the involved bone are early features of this neoplasm, with a definite history of trauma frequently preceding the onset of this tumour. Mandible is more often affected than maxilla. The radiographic findings vary from dense sclerosis to a mixed sclerotic and radiolucent lesion to an entirely radiolucent process. An important early manifestation of osteosarcoma of the jaws is the finding of a symmetrically widened periodontal ligament space about one or more teeth on the dental periapical roentgenogram.

***Histopathologic Features:*** The essential microscopic criterion is the direct production of osteoid by malignant mesenchymal cells. There is proliferation of both atypical osteoblasts and their less differentiated precursors. Vascular channels are often a common feature and a small number of multinucleated giant cells may be present.

7. **Malignant lymphoma:** The malignant lymphomas constitute a group of neoplasms of varying degrees of malignancy which are derived from the basic cells of lymphoid tissue, the lymphocytes and histiocytes in any of their developmental stages.

**Hodgkin's lymphoma:** This is considered as one of the two main types of malignant lymphoma. Hodgkin's disease is primarily one of lymph nodes and lymphoid organs. The lymph nodes of the head and neck, particularly the cervical nodes, are often the initial site of involvement. The usual presenting sign is the identification by the patient of a persistently enlarging, nontender, discrete mass or masses in one lymph node region.

***Histopathologic Features:*** Hodgkin's lymphoma is currently classified in the following manner: (a) Nodular lymphocyte-predominant Hodgkin's lymphoma, or (b) Classical Hodgkin's lymphoma (comprising five histopathologic subtypes): (i) Lymphocyte rich (ii) Nodular sclerosis, (iii) Mixed cellularity, (iv) Lymphocyte depletion, (v) Unclassifiable.

These names describe the most prominent histopathologic features of each type. The common features include effacement of the normal nodal architecture by a diffuse, often mixed, infiltrate of inflammatory cells that is interspersed with binucleated Reed-Sternberg giant cells.

**Non-Hodgkin's lymphoma:** The non-Hodgkin's lymphomas involve lymph nodes and lymphoid organs as well as extranodal tissues and organs. The lymph nodes of the head and neck are commonly involved as well as the extranodal tissues of this area. In the oral cavity, lymphoma usually appears as extra-nodal disease. The malignancy may develop in the oral soft tissues or centrally within the jaws. Soft tissue lesions appear as nontender, diffuse swellings commonly affecting the buccal vestibule, posterior hard palate, or gingiva. Lymphoma of bone may cause vague pain or discomfort, which might be mistaken for a toothache. Radiographs usually show an ill-defined or ragged radiolucency.

***Histopathologic Features:*** The non-Hodgkin's lymphomas present either a nodular or a diffuse pattern of proliferation of lymphocytic appearing cells, which show varying degrees of differentiation.

**Burkitt's lymphoma:** Also known as African jaw lymphoma this malignancy is of β-lymphocyte origin that represents an undifferentiated lymphoma. This malignancy is thought to be related pathogenetically to Epstein-Barr virus. The endemic African form of the disease is confined almost exclusively to children between 2 and 14 years of age. It is a rapidly growing tumour mass of the jaws, destroying the bone and causing loosening of the teeth with extension to involve the maxillary, ethmoid and sphenoid sinuses as well as the orbit. Radiograph shows a radiolucent destruction of the bone with ragged, ill-defined margins.

***Histopathologic Features:*** The tumour consists of a monotonous overgrowth of undifferentiated monomorphic lymphoreticular cells, usually showing abundant mitotic activity. Presence of macrophages produces a classic starry-sky pattern within the lesion where the macrophages stand out as "stars" set against the "night sky" of deeply hyperchromatic neoplastic lymphoid cells.

8. **Multiple myeloma:** Multiple myeloma is a relatively uncommon malignancy of plasma cell origin which appears to have a multicentric origin within bone. Bone pain is the most characteristic presenting symptom due to bone destruction and pathologic fractures. Jaw involvement includes pain, swelling, and expansion of the jaw, numbness and mobility of teeth. Extraosseous lesions may occur which resemble gingival enlargements. Radiographically, multiple well-defined, "punched-out" radiolucencies or ragged radiolucent lesions may be seen in multiple myeloma, which is especially evident on a skull film.

***Histopathologic Features:*** The lesion is composed of sheets of closely packed cells resembling plasma cells with variable differentiation and frequent mitotic activity. Occasionally, deposition of amyloid may be observed in association with the neoplastic cells.

Exercise Four

# TUMOURS OF THE SALIVARY GLANDS

The classification scheme of salivary gland tumours is a dynamic one that changes as clinicians learn more about these lesions. The commonly occurring tumours are:

**BENIGN:**

1. **Pleomorphic Adenoma ("Mixed Tumour"):** It is the most common of all salivary gland tumours being derived from a mixture of ductal and myoepithelial elements. Parotid gland is most commonly affected followed by submandibular gland and minor salivary glands. The pleomorphic adenoma typically appears as a painless, slow growing firm swelling which if neglected can attain grotesque proportions.

***Histopathologic Features:*** This neoplasm presents diverse histologic features, which is a characteristic finding. The encapsulated tumour is composed of a mixture of glandular epithelium and myoepithelial cells within a mesenchyme-like background. The epithelium often forms ducts and cystic structures or may occur as islands or sheets of cells. Myoepithelial cells are present with variable morphology and the characteristic "stromal" changes are believed to be produced by the myoepithelial cells. Loose myxoid material is a predominant feature, while foci of hyalinized connective tissue, or cartilage-like material and even bone, are common.

2. **Papillary Cystadenoma Lymphomatosum (Warthin's Tumour):** Warthin tumour is a benign neoplasm that occurs almost exclusively in the parotid gland. It is suggested that they arise from heterotopic salivary gland tissue found within parotid lymph nodes. The tumour is generally superficial, slow growing painless mass, which is firm to palpation and seldom exceeds 3 to 4 cm in diameter.

***Histopathologic Features:*** The tumour is composed of a mixture of ductal epithelium and a lymphoid stroma. The epithelial cells are usually arranged in two rows exhibiting papillary projections extending into cystic spaces, which frequently contain an eosinophilic coagulum. The abundant lymphoid component may represent the normal lymphoid tissue of lymph node with germinal centers.

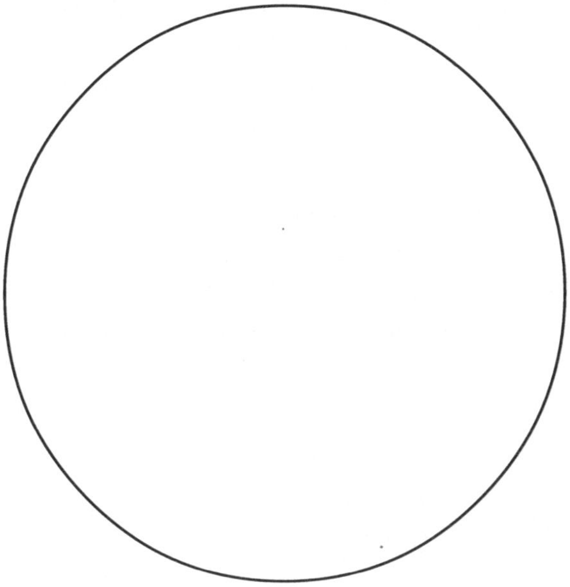

## MALIGNANT:

1. **Adenoid Cystic Carcinoma**: The adenoid cystic carcinoma is one of the more common salivary malignancies. It is also called cylindroma because of its distinctive histopathologic features. It commonly occurs within the minor salivary glands mainly affecting the palate. It usually appears as a slow-growing mass with accompanying pain, which is an early and important finding. Facial nerve paralysis may develop with parotid tumours. Tumours arising in the palate or maxillary sinus may show radiographic evidence of bone destruction.

***Histopathologic Features:*** The adenoid cystic carcinoma is composed of small, deeply staining uniform cells arranged in anastomosing cords or ductlike pattern, the central portion of which may contain a mucoid material, producing the typical cribriform or "honey-comb" pattern. The stromal connective tissue becomes hyalinized and surrounds the tumour cells, forming a structural pattern of cylinders from which the lesion originally derived the name "cylindroma".

2. **Acinic Cell Carcinoma (Adenocarcinoma):** This tumour possesses distinct clinicopathologic features and is one of the more common minor salivary gland malignancies. The tumour most often appears as a painless mass that may have been present for a long time with slow growth. Tumour can erode or infiltrate the underlying bone.
***Histopathologic Features:*** The acinic cell carcinoma, which is frequently surrounded by a thin capsule, may be composed of cells of varying degrees of differentiation. Well-differentiated cells bear remarkable resemblance to normal acinar cells; whereas less differentiated cells resemble embryonic ducts and immature acinar cells. The cells may grow in a solid pattern or form cords, ducts, or larger cystic spaces. The stroma is often mucoid in nature, or it may demonstrate hyalinization.

3. **Mucoepidermoid Carcinoma:** The mucoepidermoid carcinoma is one of the most common salivary gland malignancies. It is the most common salivary gland malignancy in children. It presents varying degrees or grades of malignancy. It is common in parotid gland and is usually asymptomatic with pain being a feature of high-grade tumours. The minor glands constitute the second most common site, especially the palate. Interosseous tumours also may develop in the jaws.

***Histopathologic Features:*** The mucoepidermoid carcinoma is composed of a mixture of mucus-producing cells, squamous (epidermoid cells) and intermediate cells. On occasion, clusters of clear cells may be present. These tumours show sheets or nests of epidermoid and mucous cells usually arranged in a glandular pattern and sometimes showing microcyst formation.

# ODONTOGENIC CYST

## ODONTOGENIC CYSTS

**Cyst:** A cyst is a pathological cavity having fluid, semifluid or gaseous contents and which is not created by the accumulation of pus (Kramer 1974). It is frequently, but not always, lined by epithelium. Other than a few cysts that may result from the inclusion of epithelium along embryonic lines of fusion, most jaw cysts are lined by epithelium that is derived from odontogenic epithelium. These are referred to as odontogenic cysts.

## Classification of Odontogenic Cysts

### DEVELOPMENTAL

1. Dentigerous cyst
2. Eruption cyst
3. Odontogenic keratocyst
4. Gingival cyst of the newborn
5. Gingival cyst of the adult
6. Lateral periodontal cyst
7. Calcifying odontogenic cyst
8. Glandular odontogenic cyst

### INFLAMMATORY

1. Radicular cyst
2. Residual cyst
3. Paradental cyst
4. Buccal bifurcation cyst

### DEVELOPMENTAL CYSTS

1. **Dentigerous cyst:** The dentigerous cyst is defined as a cyst that originates by the separation of the follicle from around the crown of an unerupted tooth. The dentigerous cyst encloses the crown of an unerupted tooth and is attached to the tooth at the cementoenamel junction. The pathogenesis of this cyst is uncertain, but apparently it develops by accumulation of fluid between the reduced enamel epithelium and the tooth crown.

***Radiographic Features:*** Radiographically the dentigerous cyst typically shows a unilocular radiolucent area that is associated with the crown of an unerupted tooth most often involving mandibular third molars. The cyst-to-crown relationship shows several radiographic variations namely, central, lateral and circumferential where the

radiolucency surrounding the crown is centrally around the crown, lateral to the crown or surrounds the crown and extends for some distance along the root.

***Histopathologic Features:*** It is usually composed of a thin connective tissue wall with a thin layer of stratified squamous epithelium lining the lumen. Rete peg formation is generally absent except in cases that are secondarily infected.

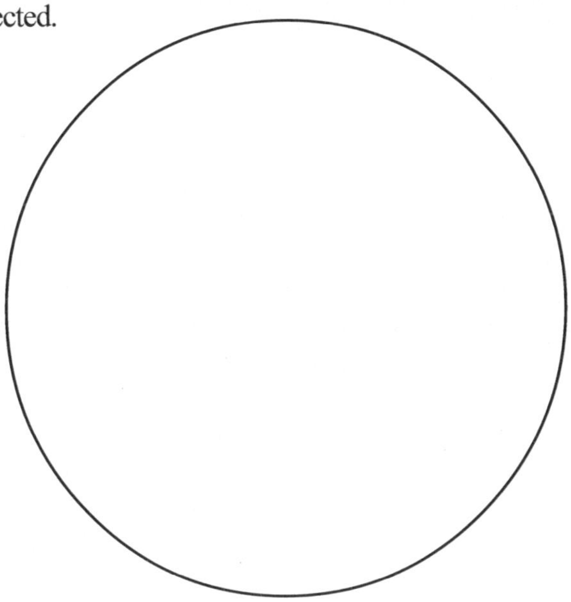

2. **Eruption cyst:** The eruption cyst is the soft tissue analogue of the dentigerous cyst. The cyst develops as a result of separation of the dental follicle from around the crown of an erupting tooth that is within the soft tissues overlying the alveolar bone. When the circumcoronal cystic cavity contains blood, the swelling appears purple or deep blue; hence the term "eruption haematoma".

***Histopathologic Features:*** Surface oral epithelium is seen on the superior aspect with a variable degree of inflammatory cell infiltrate in the underlying lamina propria. Deeper portion shows the roof of the cyst, which is composed of a thin layer of nonkeratinizing squamous epithelium.

3. **Odontogenic keratocyst:** The odontogenic keratocyst arises from cell rests of the dental lamina and has characteristic histopathologic features and clinical behaviour. The term "primordial cyst" has been synonymously used with "odontogenic keratocyst" but not all primordial cysts are odontogenic keratocysts in the original context of a primordial cyst being one developing in place of a tooth through degeneration of an enamel organ. A cyst clinically considered to represent a primordial cyst, in the older meaning of the term, almost always is an odontogenic keratocyst after microscopic study.

***Radiographic appearance:*** Odontogenic keratocysts tend to grow in an anteroposterior direction within the medullary cavity of the bone without causing obvious bone expansion. They demonstrate a well-defined radiolucent area with smooth and often corticated margins.

***Histopathologic Features:*** The odontogenic keratocyst typically shows a thin, friable wall, which is essentially devoid of any inflammatory infiltrate. The lining epithelium is highly characteristic and is composed of a parakeratin surface, which is usually corrugated. Epithelium is uniform and of 6 to10 cells layer thick without rete peg formation with a palisaded basal layer of cells. Small satellite cysts or islands of odontogenic epithelium may be seen within the fibrous wall.

4. **Gingival cyst of the newborn:** Gingival cysts of the newborn are small, superficial, keratin-filled cysts that are found on the alveolar mucosa of infants. These cysts arise from remnants of the dental lamina. Similar inclusion cysts are also found in the midline of the palate (Epstein's pearls) or laterally on the hard and soft palate (Bohn's nodules).

***Histopathologic Features:*** Examination of an intact gingival cyst of the newborn shows a thin, flattened epithelial lining with a parakeratotic surface. The lumen contains keratinaceous debris.

5. **Gingival cyst of the adult:** The gingival cyst of the adult is an uncommon lesion and is considered to represent the soft tissue counterpart of the lateral periodontal cyst being derived from rests of the dental lamina (rests of Serres). They appear as painless, domelike swellings, usually less than 0.5 cm in diameter and are often bluish or bluish-gray in colour.

***Histopathologic Features:*** The histopathologic appearance is similar to that of the lateral periodontal cyst, consisting of a thin, flattened epithelial lining with or without focal plaques that contain clear cells.

6. **Lateral periodontal cyst:** The lateral periodontal cyst is an uncommon type of developmental odontogenic cyst that typically occurs along the lateral root surface of a tooth. It is believed to arise from rests of the dental lamina and it represents the intrabony counterpart of the gingival cyst of the adult. Botryoid odontogenic cyst is the term used to designate the polycystic variant of the lateral periodontal cyst developing through cystic transformation of multiple islands of dental lamina rests.

***Radiographic appearance:*** It appears as a radiolucent area in apposition to the lateral surface of a tooth root, which is seldom over 1cm in diameter with a definitive sclerotic border.

***Histopathologic Features:*** The lateral periodontal cyst has a thin; generally non-inflamed, fibrous wall with an epithelial lining that is only 1 to 3 cells thick in most areas. Foci of glycogen-rich clear cells may be interspersed among the lining epithelial cells. Focal thickened plaques of proliferating lining cells often project into the lumen in areas.

7. **Calcifying odontogenic cyst (Gorlin cyst):** It is an uncommon lesion that demonstrates considerable histopathologic diversity and variable clinical behaviour. Different types of this cyst are classified as type 1A, the simple unicystic type; type1B, the odontome producing type; type 1C, the ameloblastomatous proliferating type, and type 2 the neoplastic type.

***Radiographic Features:*** The central intrabony lesions appear as radiolucency, usually rather well circumscribed with variable amounts of calcified radiopaque material scattered throughout the radiolucency.

***Histopathologic Features:*** Most commonly, a well-defined cystic lesion is found with a fibrous capsule and a lining of odontogenic epithelium of 4 to 10 cells in thickness. The superficial layer of epithelium is loosely arranged and may resemble the stellate reticulum of an ameloblastoma. Presence of variable numbers of ghost cells within the epithelial component is a characteristic feature of the cyst. Calcification within the ghost cells is common.

8. **Glandular odontogenic cyst (Sialo-odontogenic cyst):** The glandular odontogenic cyst is a rare and recently recognized type of developmental odontogenic cyst that can show aggressive behaviour. It shows both odontogenic and glandular or salivary features, which presumably are an indication of the pluripotentiality of odontogenic epithelium. It commonly occurs in the anterior region of the jaws.

***Radiographic Features:*** Radiographically, the lesion may appear as a unilocular or more commonly a multilocular radiolucency with well-defined margin.

***Histopathologic Features:*** The glandular odontogenic cyst is lined by squamous epithelium of varying thickness with a flat interface between the epithelium and fibrous connective tissue wall. Pools of mucin are often present within the epithelium. Mucous cells may or may not be present within the epithelium.

## INFLAMMATORY CYSTS

1. **Periapical cyst (radicular cyst):** Periapical cyst is the most common of the odontogenic cysts. It involves the apex of an erupted tooth and is most frequently a result of infection via the pulp chamber and root canal through carious involvement of the tooth. The epithelial lining is usually derived from the epithelial rests of Malassez in the periodontal ligament.

***Radiographic Features:*** There is a loss of the lamina dura along the adjacent root, and a rounded radiolucency encircles the affected tooth apex.

***Histopathologic Features:*** The cyst is lined by stratified squamous epithelium, which may demonstrate exocytosis, spongiosis, or hyperplasia. The lumen is filled with fluid and cellular debris. Occasionally, the lining epithelium may demonstrate linear or arch-shaped calcifications known as Rushton bodies. The wall of the cyst consists of dense fibrous connective tissue, with almost universal occurrence of an inflammatory infiltrate adjacent to the epithelium. This infiltrate varies in its composition but generally is made up of lymphocytes and plasma cells, with some admixed polymorphonuclear leukocytes, depending partially upon the intensity of the infection. In some lesions, collections of cholesterol slits with associated multinucleated giant cells are found in the wall of the lesion.

2. **Residual cyst:** Periapical inflammatory tissue that is not curetted at the time of tooth removal may give rise to an inflammatory cyst called a residual periapical cyst. It appears as a round-to-oval radiolucency of variable size within the alveolar ridge at the site of a previous tooth extraction.

***Histopathologic Features:*** Histopathologic features are similar to periapical cyst. With time, many of these cysts exhibit an overall reduction in size, and spontaneous resolution can occur from a lack of continued inflammatory stimulus.

3. **Paradental cyst:** The development of inflammatory cysts on the lateral aspect of a root as a consequence of an inflammatory process in a periodontal pocket is termed paradental cysts. Such lesions typically occur distal or buccal of partially erupted mandibular third molars with a history of pericoronitis. The distinction of paradental cysts from secondarily inflamed dentigerous cysts is difficult, if not impossible, in many instances.

***Histopathologic Features:*** Histologically, the cysts are lined by a hyperplastic, non-keratinized, stratified squamous epithelium. An intense inflammatory cell infiltrate is present associated with the hyperplastic epithelium and in the fibrous capsule adjacent to the epithelium.

4. **Buccal bifurcation cyst:** The buccal bifurcation cyst is an uncommon inflammatory odontogenic cyst that characteristically develops on the buccal aspect of the mandibular first permanent molar. The pathogenesis of this cyst is uncertain. It is thought that when the tooth erupts, an inflammatory response may occur in the surrounding follicular tissues that stimulate cyst formation. It typically occurs in children from 5 to 11 years of age.

***Radiographic Features:*** Radiographs typically show a well-circumscribed unilocular radiolucency involving the buccal furcation and root area of the involved tooth.

***Histopathologic Features:*** The microscopic features are nonspecific and show a cyst that is lined by nonkeratinizing stratified squamous epithelium with areas of hyperplasia. A prominent chronic inflammatory cell infiltrate is present in the surrounding connective tissue wall.

# ODONTOGENIC TUMOURS

Odontogenic tumours are a complex group of lesions with diverse histopathologic types and clinical behaviour. Some of these lesions are true neoplasms while others may represent tumourlike malformations (hamartomas).

**Classification:**

A. Tumours of odontogenic epithelium
   1. Ameloblastoma
      a. Malignant ameloblastoma
      b. Ameloblastic carcinoma
   2. Clear cell odontogenic tumour
   3. Adenomatoid odontogenic tumour
   4. Calcifying epithelial odontogenic tumour
   5. Squamous odontogenic tumour

B. Mixed odontogenic tumours
   1. Ameloblastic fibroma
   2. Ameloblastic fibro-odontoma
   3. Ameloblastic fibrosarcoma
   4. Odontoameloblastoma
   5. Compound odontoma
   6. Complex odontoma

C. Tumours of odontogenic ectomesenchyme
   1. Odontogenic fibroma
   2. Granular cell odontogenic tumour
   3. Odontogenic myxoma
   4. Cementoblastoma.

## TUMOURS OF ODONTOGENIC EPITHELIUM

1. **Ameloblastoma:** Ameloblastomas are slow growing, locally invasive odontogenic tumours which are usually unicentric, non-functional, intermittent in growth, anatomically benign and clinically persistent. It is the most common odontogenic tumour, which may arise from rests of dental lamina, from a developing enamel organ, from the epithelial lining of an odontogenic cyst, or from the basal cells of the oral mucosa. There are three different clinicoradiographic types of ameloblastoma namely:

   a. Conventional solid or multicystic (most common)
   b. Unicystic (less common).
   c. Peripheral or extraosseous (rare).

The typical ameloblastoma begins insidiously as a central lesion of bone, which is slowly destructive, but tends to expand the bone rather than perforate it.

***Radiographic Features:*** Frequently ameloblastomas show rounded, well-defined, multilocular, cyst-like radiolucent areas with well-defined margins. The lesion is often described as having a "soap bubble" or a "honeycombed" appearance. The margins of these radiolucent lesions often show irregular scalloping.

***Histopathologic Features:*** The follicular and plexiform patterns are the most common. Less common histopathologic patterns include the acanthomatous, granular cell, desmoplastic, and basal cell types.

**Follicular ameloblastoma:** Follicular ameloblastomas consist of islands or trabeculae of epithelial cells in a connective tissue stroma. These epithelial islands consist of a core of loosely arranged polygonal or angular cells, resembling stellate reticulum, surrounded by a well-organized single layer (palisade) of tall, columnar, ameloblast like cells with nuclei at the opposite pole to the basement membrane (reversed nuclear polarity).

**Plexiform ameloblastoma:** They consist largely of thin trabeculae of epithelium typically bordered by less well-differentiated columnar cells than the ameloblast-like cells of the follicular type. The supporting stroma tends to be loosely arranged and vascular.

**Malignant ameloblastoma:** The term "malignant ameloblastoma" has been defined as that particular ameloblastoma which has given evidence of truly malignant behaviour, judged chiefly by the occurrence of metastasis, but in which the metastatic lesions have shown no significant histologic differences from the primary tumour.
**Ameloblastic carcinoma:** The term "ameloblastic carcinoma" has been defined as that type of ameloblastoma in which there has been obvious histologically malignant transformation of the epithelial component. Here the metastatic tumour resembles an epidermoid carcinoma.

2. **Clear cell odontogenic tumour:** It is a rare jaw tumour, which appears to be of odontogenic origin but of uncertain histogenesis. Histochemical and ultrastructural studies show that the clear cells, which are the prominent feature of this neoplasm, have similarities to glycogen-rich presecretory ameloblastomas.

3. **Adenomatoid odontogenic tumour:** Adenomatoid odontogenic tumour is best classified as a hamartoma rather than a true neoplasm owing to its slow growth and circumscription of the lesion. It is characterized by the formation of ductlike structures by the epithelial component of the lesion. It frequently occurs in the maxilla associated with an unerupted tooth commonly the maxillary cuspid.
***Radiographic Features:*** Commonly the tumour appears as a circumscribed, unilocular radiolucency that involves the crown of an unerupted tooth, most often a canine.
***Histopathologic Features:*** The adenomatoid odontogenic tumour is composed of epithelial cells, usually with only a scanty stroma of connective tissue. The polyhedral or spindle-shaped epithelial cells are arranged in ductlike or adenomatoid fashion. The central space is empty or contains small amounts of eosinophilic material, which may stain for amyloid.
Small foci of calcification may also be scattered throughout the tumour.

4. **Calcifying epithelial odontogenic tumour (Pindborg tumour):** Pindborg tumour is an uncommon odontogenic tumour of uncertain histogenesis.
***Radiographic Features:*** The tumour shows a unilocular or more often a multilocular radiolucency containing calcified structures of varying size and density. The tumour is frequently associated with an impacted tooth, most often a mandibular third molar.

***Histopathologic Features:*** The tumour cells bear a close morphologic resemblance to the cells of the stratum intermedium of the enamel organ. It is composed of discrete islands, strands, or sheets of polyhedral epithelial cells in a fibrous stroma. The cellular outlines of the epithelial cells are distinct, and intercellular bridges may be noted. Large areas of amorphous, eosinophilic, hyalinized (amyloid-like) extracellular material are also often present. Calcifications, which are a distinctive feature of the tumour, develop within the amyloid-like material and form concentric rings (Liesegang ring calcifications). These tend to fuse together and form large, complex masses.

5. **Squamous odontogenic tumour:** Squamous odontogenic tumour is a rare benign odontogenic neoplasm which may be histologically misdiagnosed as an acanthomatous ameloblastoma or a well-differentiated squamous cell carcinoma. The tumour appears to originate within the periodontal ligament that is associated with the lateral root surface of an erupted tooth and may arise from neoplastic transformation of dental lamina rests, or the epithelial rests of malassez.

***Radiographic Features:*** The radiographic findings are not diagnostic and consist of a triangular radiolucent defect lateral to the root or roots of the teeth.

***Histopathologic Features:*** The squamous odontogenic tumour is composed of islands of mature squamous epithelium without a peripheral palisaded or polarized columnar layer. Other findings may be microcyst formation involving only small portions of the epithelial islands, laminar calcifications in the epithelium and globular, hyalin, eosinophilic structures within the islands, which are not amyloid.

## MIXED ODONTOGENIC TUMOURS

1. **Ameloblastic fibroma:** The ameloblastic fibroma is considered to be a true mixed tumour in which the epithelial and mesenchymal tissues are both neoplastic. It is suggested that the ameloblastic fibroma represents an immature complex odontoma and that, if the tumour is left undisturbed, it will ultimately differentiate or mature further into a lesion known as an ameloblastic fibro-odontoma and then continue maturation into a completely differentiated odontoma.

***Radiographic Features:*** It is manifested as a unilocular or multilocular, radiolucent lesion often with a sclerotic border.

***Histopathologic Features:*** The characteristic appearance consists of scattered islands of epithelial cells arranged in rosettes, strands or cords. The mesenchymal component is made up of a primitive connective tissue consisting of plump stellate and ovoid cells in a loose matrix, which closely resembles the developing dental papilla.

2. **Ameloblastic fibro-odontoma:** The ameloblastic fibro-odontoma has the general features of an ameloblastic fibroma but it also contains enamel and dentin. It is thought to represent an immature complex odontoma and therefore represents a hamartomatous malformation rather than a neoplastic odontogenic lesion.

***Radiographic Features:*** The lesion shows a well-circumscribed expansile radiolucency generally containing either a solitary radiopaque mass or multiple small opacities representing the odontoma portion of the lesion.

***Histopathologic Features:*** Microscopically the lesion is identical to ameloblastic fibroma and has narrow cords and islands of odontogenic epithelium in a loose primitive-appearing connective tissue that resembles dental papilla. The calcifying element consists of foci of enamel and dentin matrix formation in close relationship to the epithelial structures.

3. **Odontoma:** Odontomas are considered to be developmental anomalies (hamartomas) rather than true neoplasms. When fully developed, odontomas consist chiefly of enamel and dentin with variable amounts of pulp and cementum. This lesion is composed of more than one type of tissue and hence, called a composite odontoma. Odontomas are further subdivided into compound and complex types. The compound composite odontoma is composed of multiple, small toothlike structures and is found more often in the anterior maxilla. The complex composite odontoma consists of a conglomerate mass of enamel and dentin with no anatomic resemblance to a tooth and has a predilection to the posterior jaws.

***Radiographic Features:*** Radiographically, the compound composite odontoma appears as a collection of toothlike structures of varying size and shape surrounded by a narrow radiolucent zone. The complex composite odontoma appears as a calcified mass with the radiodensity of tooth structure, which is also surrounded by a narrow radiolucent rim.

***Histopathologic Features:*** Histologically, normal-appearing enamel or enamel matrix, dentin, pulp tissue and cementum are found which may or may not exhibit a normal relation to one another. The connective tissue capsule around the odontoma is similar in all respects to the follicle surrounding a normal tooth.

## TUMOURS OF ODONTOGENIC ECTOMESENCHYME

1. **Odontogenic fibroma:** The odontogenic fibromas may be central (intraosseous) or peripheral. These are uncommon and somewhat controversial lesions.

***Radiographic Features:*** Radiographically, the central odontogenic fibromas tend to be well-defined, unilocular, radiolucent lesions often associated with the periradicular area of erupted tooth. Larger lesions tend to be multilocular radiolucencies.

***Histopathologic Features:*** The peripheral odontogenic fibroma consists of a markedly cellular fibrous connective tissue parenchyma with non-neoplastic islands of odontogenic epithelium. The central odontogenic fibroma is composed of stellate fibroblasts often arranged in a whorled pattern with fine collagen fibrils and considerable ground substance. Small foci of odontogenic epithelial rests may or may not be present. Occasionally foci of dystrophic calcifications may be present.

2. **Odontogenic myxoma:** Myxomas of the jaws are believed to arise from odontogenic ectomesenchyme. They resemble the mesenchymal portion of a developing tooth.

***Radiographic Features:*** The myxoma appears as a unilocular or multilocular radiolucency that may displace or cause resorption of teeth in the area of the tumour. Large myxomas of the mandible may show a "soap-bubble" radiolucent pattern.

***Histopathologic Features:*** Gross examination of myxoma reveals a loose gelatinous structure. Microscopically the tumour is composed of haphazardly arranged stellate, spindle-shaped, and round cells in an abundant, loose myxoid stroma that contains only a few collagen fibrils. Histochemical study shows that the ground substance is composed of glycosaminoglycans, chiefly hyaluronic acid and chondroitin sulphate.

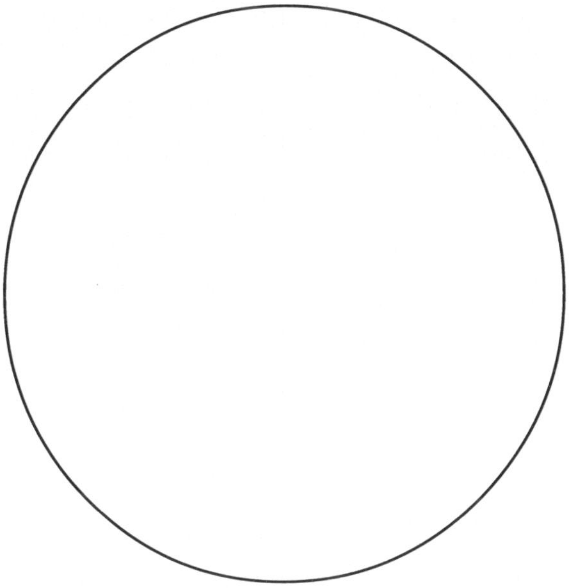

3. **Benign cementoblastoma (true cementoma):** Cementoblastoma is an odontogenic neoplasm of cementoblasts which is believed to be the only true neoplasm of cementum. Functional cementoblasts form a large

mass of cementum or cementum-like tissue on the tooth root. It is a rare odontogenic neoplasm occurring in the age group under 25 years and more common in the mandible.

***Radiographic Features:*** The tumour appears as a radiopaque mass that is fused to one or more tooth roots and is surrounded by a thin radiolucent rim.

***Histopathologic Features:*** The histopathologic appearance of cementoblastoma closely resembles that of osteoblastoma, with the main differentiating feature being tumour fusion with the involved tooth. The main bulk of the tumour mass is composed of sheets of cementum-like tissue with irregularly placed lacunae and prominent basophilic reversal lines. The periphery of the mass is composed of uncalcified matrix, which often is arranged in radiating columns.

Exercise Seven

# BACTERIAL, VIRAL AND FUNGAL INFECTIONS

Certain bacteria, viruses and fungi produce diseases, which are manifested in or about the oral cavity.

**Bacterial infections:**

1. Scarlet fever
2. Diphtheria
3. Tuberculosis
4. Sarcoidosis
5. Leprosy
6. Actinomycosis
7. Syphilis
8. Gonorrhoea
9. Wegener's granulomatosis
10. Pyogenic granuloma

**Viral infections:**

1. Herpes simplex
2. Recurrent aphthous stomatitis
3. Herpangina
4. Hand, foot and mouth disease
5. Measles
6. Smallpox
7. Chickenpox
8. Herpes zoster
9. Mumps
10. Cytomegalic inclusion disease

**Fungal infections:**

1. Histoplasmosis
2. Coccidioidomycosis
3. Cryptococcosis
4. Candidiasis
5. Geotrichosis
6. Phycomycosis
7. Sporotrichosis
8. Rhinosporidiosis

1. **Tuberculosis:** Tuberculosis is an infectious granulomatous disease caused by the acid-fast bacillus mycobacterium tuberculosis. Typically the patients have a low-grade fever, malaise, anorexia, weight loss, and night sweats. The most common extrapulmonary site in the head and neck are the cervical lymph nodes. Tuberculous lesions are relatively uncommon in the oral cavity. Tongue, palate, lips, buccal mucosa and gingiva may be affected. The usual tuberculous lesion is an irregular, superficial or deep, painful ulcer, which tends to increase slowly in size. Tuberculosis may also involve the bone of the maxilla or mandible, which may be as tuberculous periapical granuloma or diffuse involvement by hematogenous spread.

***Histopathologic Features:*** Areas of infection demonstrate foci of caseous necrosis surrounded by epithelioid cells, lymphocytes and occasional multinucleated Langhan's type giant cells. Diagnosis can be confirmed only by demonstration of the organisms in the lesion, coupled with culture and animal inoculation.

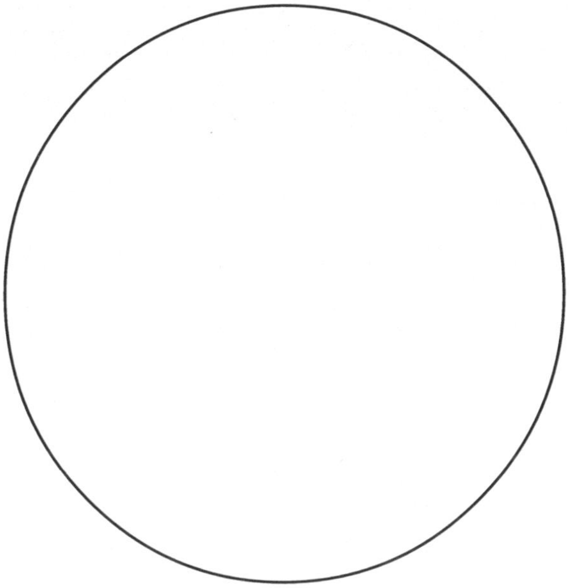

2. **Actinomycosis:** It is an infection of filamentous, branching, gram-positive anaerobic bacteria, the most commonly isolated organism being Actinomyces Israeli. Cervicofacial actinomycosis is the most common form of this disease and is characterized by formation of a "wooden" indurated area of fibrosis, which ultimately forms a central, softer area of abscess. The infection may extend to the surface, forming a sinus tract, liberating pus containing typical "sulphur granules".

***Histopathologic Features:*** The tissue demonstrates a peripheral band of fibrosis encasing a zone of chronically inflamed granulation tissue surrounding large collections of polymorph nuclear leucocytes and colonies of organisms. The colonies consist of club-shaped filaments that form a radiating rosette pattern described as "ray-fungus". The central core of the colonies stains basophilic while the peripheral portion stains eosinophilic with H&E stain.

3. **Syphilis (Lues):** Syphilis is a chronic infection produced by Treponema pallidum. The disease proceeds through three stages: Primary, Secondary and Tertiary. Transmission of the disease from mother to foetus gives rise to congenital syphilis.

*Primary syphilis* characterized by chancre. The oral lesion appears as a painless, clean-based ulceration most commonly occurring on the lip followed by tongue, palate, gingiva and tonsils.

*Secondary syphilis* discovered clinically 4 to10 weeks after the initial infection. Focal areas of intense exocytosis and spongiosis of the oral mucosa, leading to zones of sensitive whitish mucosa occur known as mucous patches.

*Tertiary syphilis* symptom-free stage called latent syphilis, which may last from 1 to 30 years. Characteristic scattered foci of granulomatous inflammation affect the skin, mucosa, soft tissue, bones and internal organs called gumma. Intraoral lesions usually affect the palate or tongue.

*Congenital syphilis* the three pathognomonic diagnostic features known as Hutchinson's triad are:

1. Hutchinson's teeth
2. Ocular interstitial keratosis
3. Eighth nerve deafness

What are mulberry molars?

Describe Hutchinson's incisors.

Enumerate the generalized features of congenital syphilis.

***Histopathologic Features:*** The histopathologic picture of oral lesions is non-specific. Oral tertiary lesions typically exhibit surface ulceration, with peripheral pseudoepitheliomatous hyperplasia. The underlying inflammatory infiltrate usually demonstrates foci of granulomatous inflammation with well-circumscribed collections of histiocytes and multinucleated giant cells.

4. **Pyogenic granuloma:** It is a distinctive clinical entity originating as a response of the tissues to a nonspecific infection. Recently it is thought to represent an exuberant tissue response to local irritation or trauma. It appears as a smooth or lobulated mass of high vascularity occurring on the gingiva, lips, tongue or buccal mucosa.

***Histopathologic Features:*** Histologically it is similar to that of granulation tissue but is exuberant and usually well localized. The surface is usually ulcerated and replaced by a thick fibrinopurulent membrane. The occurrence of vast numbers of endothelium-lined vascular spaces and extreme proliferation of fibroblasts and budding endothelial cells are prominent features. A mixed inflammatory cell infiltrate of neutrophils, plasma cells, and lymphocytes is evident.

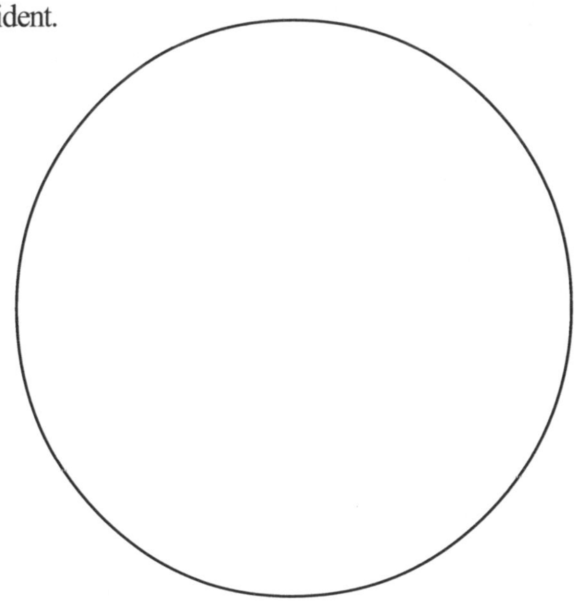

5. **Herpes simplex:** Herpes simplex is the most common acute infectious disease of viral origin. Immunologically there are two types of HSV: type 1 and type 2.
*HSV type1:* Affects the face, lips, oral cavity and upper body skin.
*HSV type 2:* Usually affects the genitals and skin of the lower body.
The affected mucosa develops numerous pinhead vesicles, which rapidly collapse to form numerous small, red lesions. The lesions may subside within 7 to 14 days.
***Histopathologic Features:*** The herpetic vesicle is an intraepithelial blister filled with fluid. Degenerating cells show "ballooning degeneration". The acantholytic epithelial cells are called Tzanck cells. Cells may contain intra-nuclear inclusions known as Lipschutz bodies. Nucleolar fragmentation occurs with a condensation of chromatin around the periphery of the nucleus. The subjacent connective tissue is usually infiltrated by inflammatory cells.

6. **Recurrent aphthous stomatitis:** It is a common disease of debatable etiology characterized by the development of painful, recurring solitary or multiple ulcerations of the oral mucosa. The lesions are similar to herpetic gingivostomatitis. The three clinical variations of aphthous stomatitis are: (1) Minor, (2) Major, and (3) Herpetiform.The lesion begins as a single or multiple superficial erosion covered by a gray membrane with a well-circumscribed margin and surrounded by an erythematous halo. They generally persist for 7 to 14 days.

Differentiate clinically between the different types of aphthous ulcers.

***Histopathologic Features:*** The early ulcerative lesions demonstrate a central zone of ulceration, which is covered by a fibrinopurulent membrane. Deep to the area of ulceration, the connective tissue exhibits an increased vascularity and a mixed inflammatory cellular infiltrate. Anitschkow cells are seen which consist of cells with elongated nuclei containing a linear bar of chromatin with radiating processes of chromatin extending toward the nuclear membrane.

7. **Measles:** Measles is an acute, contagious, dermatropic viral infection, primarily affecting children and occurring frequently in epidemic form.
Describe the clinical features of measles.

What are Koplik's spots? Describe them.

8. **Herpes zoster:** Name the virus causing this disease.

Which other disease does this virus cause?
Herpes zoster may involve the face by infection of the trigeminal nerve. Oral mucosal lesions are common and extremely painful vesicles appear on the buccal mucosa, tongue, uvula, larynx and pharynx. Characteristic feature of the disease is the unilaterality of the lesions.
Cytologic smears reveal multinucleated giant cell (Tzanck cells) and intranuclear inclusions.

9. **Candidiasis:** Infection with the yeastlike fungal organism is termed candidiasis commonly caused by the species C. albicans. It is the most opportunistic infection in the world. Candidiasis of the oral mucosa may exhibit a variety of clinical patterns.

Classify oral candidiasis.

What is thrush?

***Histopathologic Features:*** On staining with the periodic acid-schiff (PAS) method, the candidal hyphae and yeasts can be readily identified. The organisms are easily identified by the bright magenta colour imparted by the stain. The candidal hyphae are embedded in the parakeratin layer and rarely penetrate into the viable cell layers of the epithelium unless the patient is extremely immunocompromised.

10. **Aspergillosis:** Aspergillosis is a fungal disease that is characterized by noninvasive and invasive forms. Patients with uncontrolled diabetes mellitus are susceptible to Aspergillus infections. Immunocompromised patients are particularly susceptible to oral aspergillosis and the portal of entry may be the marginal gingiva and gingival sulcus. Painful gingival ulcerations are initially noted and peripherally the mucosa and soft tissue develops diffuse swelling with a grey or violaceous hue.

***Histopathologic Features:*** Aspergillus lesions show varying numbers of branching, septate hyphae, which show a tendency to branch at an acute angle and to invade adjacent small blood vessels. Occlusion of the vessels often results in the characteristic pattern of necrosis associated with this disease.

Exercise Eight

# DENTAL CARIES

Dental caries is a microbial disease of the calcified tissues of the teeth, characterized by demineralization of the inorganic portion and destruction of the organic substance of the tooth.

**Essential factors in dental caries etiology**

**1. TOOTH**
Age
Fluorides
Morphology
Nutrition
Trace Elements
Carbonate Level

**2. FLORA**
Strep, Mutans (Substrate)
Oral Hygiene
Fluoride in Plaque

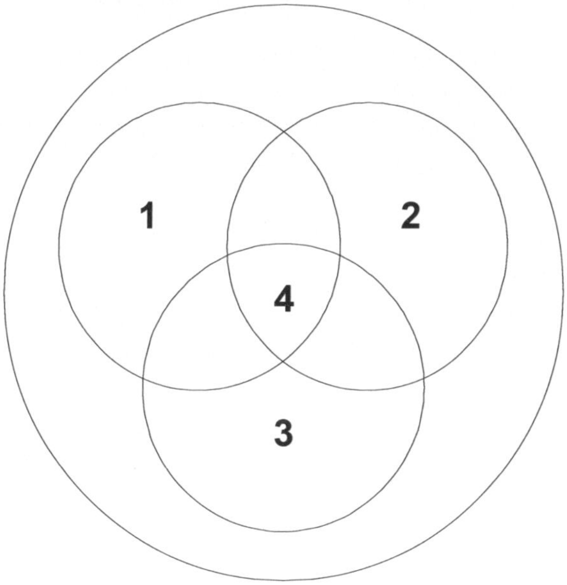


**3. SUBSTRATE**
Oral Clearance
Oral Hygiene
Salivary Stimulants
Frequency of Eating
Carbohydrate (type, concentration)

**4. CARIES**

Enumerate the theories for the etiology of dental caries.

Classify dental caries clinically.

***Histopathologic Features:*** Smooth surface caries and pit and fissure caries have different shapes of progression of caries but the zones in enamel and dentin are similar.

Name the Histologic zones of enamel caries.

Name the Histologic zones of dentinal caries.

| | | |
|---|---|---|
| Changes in enamel | : | Loss of inter-prismatic substance of enamel with increased prominence of the rods. |
| | : | Appearance of transverse striations of the enamel rods. |
| | : | Accentuation of striae of Retzius. |
| | : | Disintegration of enamel follows. |

| | | |
|---|---|---|
| Changes in dentin | : | Spread of caries process along DEJ. |
| | : | Dentinal sclerosis. |

: Appearance of fatty degeneration of Tomes' dentinal fibers.
: Bacterial invasion of dentinal tubules.
: Decalcification of dentine.

*Root caries:* A soft, progressive lesion that is found anywhere on the root surface that has lost connective tissue attachment and is exposed to the oral environment. Dental plaque and microbial invasion are an essential part of the cause and progression of this lesion.

What are the organisms responsible for root caries?

**Methods of caries control:** Classified into three general types:

1. Chemical measures
2. Nutritional measures
3. Mechanical measures

*Chemical measures include*: Fluoride, chlorhexidine, silver nitrate, zinc chloride and potassium ferro cyanide.
Enumerate the different forms of fluoride application.

*Nutritional measures include*: Restriction of refined carbohydrate intake in the diet, inclusion of phosphates in diet, vitamin K, ammonium compounds, chlorophyll, penicillin and other antibiotics.

*Mechanical measures include:* Prophylaxis by the dental professional, toothbrushing, mouth rinsing, and use of dental floss or toothpicks and incorporation of detergent foods in the diet.
Write a short note on caries vaccine.

What are caries activity tests? Name some caries activity tests.

Exercise Nine

# DISEASES OF THE DENTAL PULP

The initial response of the dental pulp to injury is similar to that seen in other tissues but the final result is different because of the rigid dentinal walls of the pulp chamber. Dental pulp is unusually fragile and sensitive because its hard dentinal casing does not allow for the usual swelling associated with the exudate of the acute inflammatory process. Moreover there is no collateral circulation to maintain vitality when the primary blood supply is compromised. Pain or increasing levels of sensitivity are the only signs that can be used to determine the severity of pulpal inflammation. The four common causes of pulpal inflammation are: mechanical damage, thermal injury, chemical irritation and bacterial effects.

**Focal reversible pulpitis:** Also referred to as pulp hyperemia, is early mild transient pulpitis, localized chiefly to the pulpal ends of irritated dentinal tubules.

What are the clinical features of focal reversible pulpitis?

***Histopathologic Features:*** Microscopically the predominant feature is dilation and engorgement of blood vessels (hyperemia), oedema and a chronic inflammatory cellular infiltrate underlying the area of affected dentinal tubules.

**Acute pulpitis:** The inflammatory response of acute pulpitis may occur as a progression of focal reversible pulpitis, or it may represent an acute exacerbation of an already established chronic pulpitis.

***Histopathologic Features:*** Acute inflammatory process spreads to involve most of the pulp. Pulpal damage may range in severity from simple acute inflammation marked by vessel dilation, exudation, and neutrophil chemotaxis to focal liquefaction necrosis (pulp abscess) to total pulpal superlative necrosis.

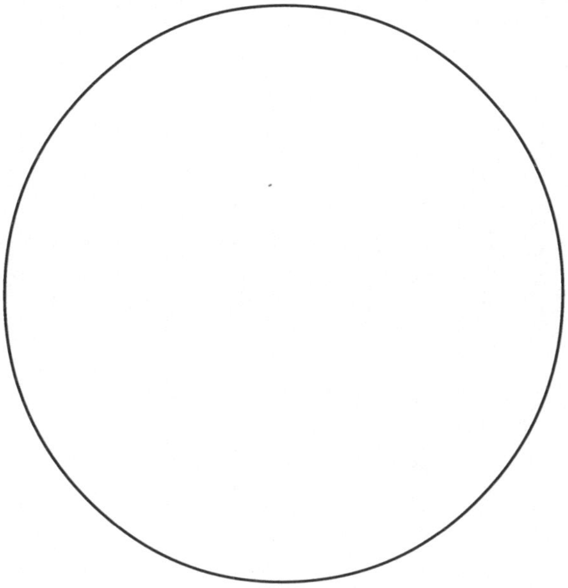

**Chronic pulpitis:** Chronic pulpitis is an inflammatory reaction that results from long-term, low-grade injury or occasionally from quiescence of an acute process. As in most chronic inflammatory conditions, the signs and symptoms are considerably milder than those in the acute form of the disease.

***Histopathologic Features:*** Microscopically, lymphocytes, plasma cells, and fibrosis appear in the chronically inflamed pulp.

**Chronic hyperplastic pulpitis (pulp polyp):** This unique form of pulpal inflammation occurs in children and young adults who have large exposures of the pulp in which the entire dentinal roof often is missing. The most frequently involved teeth are the deciduous or succedaneous molars, which have large pulp chambers in these age groups. A pulp so affected appears as a pinkish-red globule of tissue protruding from the pulp chamber and often filling the entire cavity. This type of reaction is believed to be related to the open root foramen through which relatively rich blood supply flows.

***Histopathologic Features:*** The hyperplastic tissue is basically granulation tissue made up of delicate connective tissue fibers interspersed with variable numbers of small capillaries and chronic inflammatory cell infiltration. The surface of the polyp may or may not be covered with stratified squamous epithelium, which migrates from the adjacent gingiva or arises from sloughed epithelium within the oral fluids.

# DISEASES OF THE PERIAPICAL TISSUES

Once infection has become established in the dental pulp, spread of the process takes place through the root canals and into the periapical region. Depending upon the virulence of the microorganisms involved and the integrity of the patient's overall defense mechanisms a number of different tissue reactions may occur.

**Periapical granuloma (Apical periodontitis):** The periapical granuloma is one of the most common of all sequelae of pulpitis. It is a localized mass of chronic granulation tissue at the apex of a nonvital tooth. Periapical granulomas may arise after quiescence of a periapical abscess or may develop as the initial periapical pathosis. These lesions may transform into periapical cysts or may demonstrate acute exacerbations with abscess formation. There is hyperemia, edema and inflammation of the apical periodontal ligament.
***Radiographic Features:*** It appears as a radiolucent area of variable size seemingly attached to the root apex, which may be surrounded by a sclerotic border.
***Histopathologic Features:*** Periapical granulomas consist of inflamed granulation tissue surrounded by a fibrous connective tissue wall. There is proliferation of both fibroblasts and endothelial cells and the formation of more tiny vascular channels as well as numerous delicate connective tissue fibrils. Infiltration of macrophages, lymphocytes, and plasma cells qualify it as an immune-type granuloma. Russell bodies and pyronine bodies may be present.

**Periapical cyst:** Epithelium at the apex of a non-vital tooth can be stimulated by inflammation to form a true epithelium-lined cyst, or periapical cyst. The source of the epithelium is usually a rest of Malassez but also may be traced to reticular epithelium, sinus lining, or epithelial lining of fistulous tracts.

As covered under **Cysts**:

**Periapical abscess:** The periapical abscess is an acute or chronic supportive process of the dental periapical region. Acute inflammatory lesions with abscess formation may arise as the initial periapical pathosis or from an acute exacerbation (phoenix abscess) of a chronic inflammatory periapical lesion. Periapical abscesses become symptomatic as the purulent material accumulates within the alveolus.

***Histopathologic Features:*** The area of suppuration is composed chiefly of a sea of polymorphonuclear leukocytes intermixed with inflammatory exudates, cellular debris, necrotic material, bacterial colonies or histiocytes.

**Osteomyelitis:** Osteomyelitis is the inflammation of the bone and bone marrow. In the jaws osteomyelitis may develop as a result of odontogenic infection, physical injury or even bacteremia. The disease may be acute, subacute, or chronic and presents variable clinical course depending upon its nature.

**Acute suppurative osteomyelitis:** Acute suppurative osteomyelitis of the jaw is a serious sequela of periapical infection that often results in a diffuse spread of infection throughout the medullary spaces, with subsequent necrosis of a variable amount of bone.

**Chronic suppurative osteomyelitis:** Chronic suppurative osteomyelitis may develop after the acute phase of the disease has subsided, or occasionally it may arise from a dental infection without a preceding acute stage.

**Chronic focal sclerosing osteomyelitis (condensing osteitis):** It is an unusual reaction to infection, occurring in instances of extremely high tissue resistance or in cases of a low-grade infection.

**Chronic diffuse sclerosing osteomyelitis:** It represents an inflammatory reaction in the mandible or maxilla, believed to be in response to a microorganism of low virulence. Chronic periodontal disease is important in the etiology and progression of diffuse sclerosing osteomyelitis. It tends to occur most often in middle-aged black women. The disease is characterized by a protracted chronic course with acute exacerbations of pain, swelling, and occasionally drainage.

***Radiographic Features:*** This radiopaque lesion may be extensive and is sometimes bilateral. The pattern is similar to that of the jaws in Paget's disease, which is described as having a "cotton-wool" appearance.

***Histopathologic Features:*** The microscopic changes of this condition are inflammatory. Fibrous replacement of marrow is noted. Bony trabeculae exhibit irregular size and shape and may be lined by numerous osteoblasts. The characteristic sclerotic masses are composed of dense bone, often exhibiting numerous reversal lines.

**Chronic osteomyelitis with proliferative periostitis (Garre's osteomyelitis):** Garre's osteomyelitis. It essentially is a subtype of osteomyelitis that has a prominent periosteal inflammatory reaction as an additional component. It most often results from a periapical abscess of a mandibular molar tooth or an infection associated with tooth extraction of partially erupted molars. It is most common in children.

***Radiographic Features:*** The lesion appears centrally as a mottled, predominantly lucent lesion in a pattern consistent with that of chronic osteomyelitis. Its feature that provides the distinctive difference is the periosteal reaction. This, best viewed on an occlusal radiograph, appears as an expanded cortex, often with concentric or parallel radiopaque layers. Trabeculae perpendicular to the onion skin layers may also be apparent. An occlusal X-ray shows a focal overgrowth of bone on the outer surface of the cortex, which may be described as a duplication of the cortical layer of bone.

***Histopathologic Features:*** Reactive new bone typifies the subperiosteal cortical response. Perpendicular orientation of new trabeculae to redundant cortical bone is best seen under low magnification. Osteoblastic activity dominates in this area, and both osteoblastic and osteoclastic activity are seen centrally. Marrow spaces contain fibrous tissue with scattered lymphocytes and plasma cells.

**Exercise Eleven**

# ORAL LESIONS CAUSED BY INJURIES

**Traumatic ulcer:** The traumatic ulcer of the oral mucosa may arise as a result of injury in various forms namely, biting the mucosa, denture irritation, toothbrush injury, exposure of the mucous membrane to a sharp tooth or carious lesion, or it may be injury to the mucosa by some other external irritant. They may arise on lateral border of tongue, buccal mucosa, lips or occasionally the palate.

***Histopathologic Features:*** The traumatic ulcer is a nonspecific ulcer and microscopically shows loss of continuity of surface epithelium with a fibrinous exudate covering the exposed connective tissue. The epithelium bordering the ulcer usually demonstrates proliferative activity. There is infiltration of polymorphonuclear leucocytes in the connective tissue, particularly beneath the area of ulceration, although in chronic lesions these may be replaced by lymphocytes and plasma cells. Capillary dilatation and proliferation may also be evident.

**Epulis fissuratum (Denture injury tumour):** The most common tissue reaction to a chronically ill-fitting denture is the occurrence of hyperplasia of tissue along the denture borders.

***Histopathologic Features:*** Hyperorthokeratotic or hyperparakeratotic stratified squamous epithelium with acanthosis and often showing pseudoepitheliomatous hyperplasia is seen along with a bulk of hyperplastic fibrous connective tissue composed of coarse bundles of collagen fibres with few fibroblasts or blood vessels. Mucopolysaccharide keratin dystrophy or "plasma pooling" is often seen in the surface epithelium of inflammatory fibrous hyperplasia, which consists histologically of homogeneous, eosinophilic pools of material in the superficial spinous layer of epithelium, where it appears to have replaced individual cells.

**Inflammatory papillary hyperplasia:** It is an unusual condition involving the mucosa of the palate. The exact pathogenesis of this condition is unknown but may be associated with ill-fitting dentures, poor denture hygiene or wearing of dentures for 24 hours a day. It occurs on the hard palate beneath a denture base. The mucosa is erythematous and has a pebbly or papillary surface.

***Histopathologic Features:*** The mucosa exhibits numerous papillary growths on the surface that are covered by hyperplastic stratified squamous epithelium. Pseudoepitheliomatous hyperplasia may be present. The connective tissue varies from loose and oedematous to densely collagenized. Chronic inflammatory infiltrate is usually present and underlying salivary glands if present may show metaplastic changes and sialadenitis.

**Mucocoele (Mucous extravasation phenomenon):** The traumatic severance of a salivary gland excretory duct results in mucus escape into the surrounding connective tissue resulting in an inflammatory reaction and granulation tissue forming a wall around the mucin pool. They typically appear as dome-shaped mucosal swellings that may range from 1 or 2 mm to several cms in size.

***Histopathologic Features:*** The mucocoele shows an area of spilled mucin surrounded by a wall of granulation tissue. Inflammatory response includes numerous foamy histiocytes (macrophages). The adjacent minor salivary glands often contain a chronic inflammatory cell infiltrate and dilated ducts.

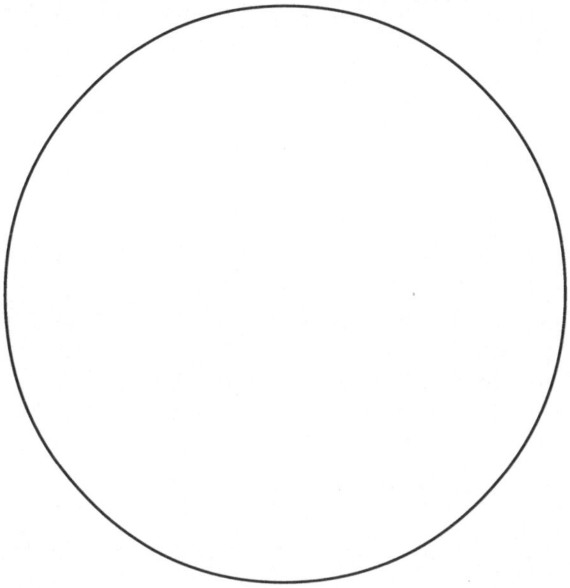

**Mucus retention cyst:** Mucus retention cyst results from obstruction of salivary flow. Unlike the more common mucocoele, it is a true cyst because it is lined by epithelium.

***Histopathologic Features:*** The cyst like cavity of a mucus retention cyst is lined by normal but compressed ductal epithelial cells varying from cuboidal, columnar, or atrophic squamous epithelium. The connective tissue around the lesion is minimally inflamed, although the associated gland shows obstructive change.

**Ranula:** Ranula is a term used for mucocoeles that occur in the floor of the mouth. The name is derived from the Latin word rana, which means frog, because the swelling may resemble a frog's translucent underbelly. Ranula is associated with the sublingual or submandibular glands and presents as a fluctuant, unilateral soft tissue mass often exhibiting a bluish colour. A deep so-called plunging ranula develops if mucus herniates through the mylohyoid muscle and along the fascial planes of the neck.

***Histopathologic Features:*** The microscopic appearance is similar to that of mucocoele except that a definite epithelial lining is sometimes present. The spilled mucin elicits a granulation tissue response that typically contains foamy histiocytes.

**Retention cyst of maxillary sinus:** Mucocoele of the maxillary antrum is an uncommon variant of the mucus retention phenomenon. It represents a retention phenomenon of the mucous glands associated with the lining of the maxillary sinus. Traumatic injury associated with tooth extraction may be of etiologic significance. It is mostly asymptomatic and is discovered only during routine radiographic examination of the jaws.

***X-ray Features:*** The lesion appears as a well-defined, homogeneous, dome-shaped or hemispheric radiopacity arising from the floor of the antrum and superimposed on it.

***Histopathologic Features:*** It consists of fluid accumulation within connective tissue spaces and have no definite lining. This type is sometimes referred to as a non-secretory cyst. Sometimes the lesion may be lined by a respiratory type of epithelium, and is described as the secretory type of antral cyst. Inflammatory cell infiltration in the connective tissue wall is common.

## Chemical Injuries

Name some drugs and chemicals, which have harmful effect on the oral mucosa.

## Wound Healing

What are the factors affecting healing of oral wounds?

## Biopsy

Define biopsy. What are the different types of biopsy?

What is exfoliative cytology? What are the grades of exfoliative cytology?

What are the stages of healing of extraction socket?

What is dry socket?

**Exercise Twelve**

# THE AVITAMINOSES

What are the oral manifestations of vitamin A deficiency?

What are the oral manifestations of vitamin D deficiency?

Describe the oral manifestations of vitamin C deficiency.

Describe the oral manifestations of vitamin B complex deficiency.

**Exercise Thirteen**

# ENDOCRINE DISTURBANCES

Name some oral manifestations of hypo and hyperpituitarism.

Name some oral manifestations of hypo and hyperthyroidism.

**Hyperparathyroidism:** Excess production of parathyroid hormone (PTH) results in the condition known as hyperparathyroidism. Primary hyperparathyroidism is the uncontrolled production of PTH usually as a result of a parathyroid adenoma or hyperplasia. Secondary hyperparathyroidism develops when PTH is continuously produced in response to chronic low levels of serum calcium, a situation usually associated with chronic renal disease. Women have this condition more often than men. The classic triad of signs and symptoms consist of renal stones, osseous changes in bones and tendency for the development of duodenal ulcers.

***Radiographic Features:*** Generalized loss of the lamina dura around teeth is an early manifestation. Alterations in trabecular patterns giving a ground glass appearance.

**Brown tumour of hyperparathyroidism:** Why is the lesion called brown tumour?

***Osteitis fibrosa cystica*** develops from the central degeneration and fibrosis of longstanding brown tumours. These lesions appear as well-demarcated unilocular or multilocular radiolucencies.

***Histopathologic Features:*** The brown tumour is histologically identical to central giant cell granuloma of the jaws. Proliferation of exceedingly vascular granulation tissue with numerous multinucleated osteoclast-type giant cells is seen.

What are the oral manifestations of diabetes mellitus?

**Exercise Fourteen**

# DISEASES OF THE BONE

Diseases of the bone constitute a group of generalized skeletal diseases which frequently manifest involvement of the maxilla or mandible.

**Osteogenesis Imperfecta:** Osteogenesis imperfecta represents a genetically heterogeneous group of heritable defects of connective tissue. Classically this condition may include fragile bones, blue sclerae, ligament laxity, hearing loss, and dentinogenesis imperfecta. Abnormal collegenous maturation results in bone with a thin cortex, fine trabeculation, and diffuse osteoporosis.

***Histopathologic Features:*** Cortical bone appears attenuated. Osteoblasts are present, but bone matrix production is reduced markedly. The bone architecture remains immature throughout life, and there is a failure of woven bone to become transformed to lamellar bone.

**Cleidocranial Dysplasia:** This is a disorder of bone caused by a defect in the CBFA 1 gene of chromosome 6p21 which normally guides osteoblastic differentiation and appropriate bone formation. Cleidocranial dysplasia is notable for aplasia or hypoplasia of the clavicles, characteristic craniofacial malformations, and the presence of numerous supernumerary and unerupted teeth.

Enumerate the craniofacial malformations noted in cleidocranial dysplasia.

What are the oral manifestations seen in cleidocranial dysplasia?

**Pierre Robin Syndrome:** What are the characteristic features of this anomalad?

Name the syndrome caused by trisomy 21. Enumerate the characteristic features of this syndrome.

**Osteopetrosis (Marble Bone Disease):** Osteopetrosis is a group of rare hereditary skeletal disorders characterized by a marked increase in bone density resulting from a defect in remodelling caused by failure of normal osteoclast function. Defective osteoblastic bone resorption, combined with continued bone formation and endochondral ossification, results in thickening of cortical bone and sclerosis of the cancellous bone.

***Radiographic Features:*** It is characterized by a diffuse, homogeneous, symmetrically sclerotic appearance of all bones with clubbing and transverse striations of the ends of the long bones. The medullary cavities are replaced by bone, and the cortex is thickened.

***Histopathologic Features:*** The pattern of endochondral bone formation is disrupted, with a decrease in osteoblastic function and a compensatory increase in the number of osteoclasts.

**Paget's Disease of Bone (Osteitis Deformans):** It is a chronic, slowly progressive bone condition of undetermined cause. Paget's disease generally progresses through several stages that include an initial resorptive phase, followed by a vascular phase, and eventually a sclerosing phase.
Describe the oral manifestations of Paget's disease.

***Roentgenographic Features:*** The early stages of Paget's disease reveal a decreased radiodensity of the bone and alteration of the trabecular pattern. The classic radiographic findings in the late stage of Paget's disease are due to bony sclerosis providing a patchy radiopaque pattern described as resembling cotton wool.
***Histopathologic Features:*** Microscopic examination shows an apparent uncontrolled alternating resorption and formation of bone. In the initial resorptive phase, random overactive osteoclastic bone resorption is evident. Resorbed bone is replaced by vascularized connective tissue along with prominent osteolysis and osteogenesis. Bone eventually develops a dense mosaic pattern as a result of reversal lines in increasingly sclerotic bone, as osteoclasts give way to osteoblasts.

**Fibrous Dysplasia of Bone:** It is a lesion of unknown etiology, uncertain pathogenesis and diverse histopathology. In this condition normal medullary bone is replaced by an abnormal fibrous connective tissue proliferation in which new, nonmaturing bone is formed.

What are the types of fibrous dysplasia? Write the features of each.

***Radiographic Features:*** Fibrous dysplasia has a variable radiographic appearance that ranges from a radiolucent lesion to a uniformly radiopaque mass. The classic design has been described as having a radiopaque change that imparts a "ground glass" or "peau d'orange" effect.

***Histopathologic Features:*** The typical microscopic findings of fibrous dysplasia show irregularly shaped trabeculae of immature (woven) bone in a cellular, loosely arranged fibrous stroma.

The bony trabeculae are not connected to each other and assume irregular shapes likened to Chinese characters, and they do not display any functional orientation.

**Cherubism:** Cherubism is a benign hereditary condition of the maxilla and/or mandible, usually found in children by 5 years of age. The cherub like facies arises from bilateral involvement of the posterior mandible that produces angelic chubby cheeks. In addition, there is an "eyes upturned to heaven" appearance that is due to a wide rim of exposed sclerae noted below the iris.

Describe the oral manifestations and radiographic appearance of cherubism.

***Histopathologic Features:*** Histologically, the lesions are composed of a vascularized fibrous stroma containing multinucleated giant cells. A characteristic feature that is often present is eosinophilic perivascular cuffing of collagen surrounding small capillaries throughout the lesion.

**Exercise Fifteen**

# DISEASES OF THE TEMPOROMANDIBULAR JOINT

**Developmental disturbances of TMJ**

- Aplasia
- Hypoplasia
- Hyperplasia
- Describe the clinical features of condylar hypoplasia.

**Traumatic disturbances of TMJ**

**Luxation and subluxation:** Dislocation of the TMJ occurs when the head of the condyle moves anteriorly over the articular eminence into such a position that it cannot be returned voluntarily to its normal position.

Describe the features of TMJ dislocation.

**Ankylosis:** Ankylosis or fusion of TMJ can be fibrous or bony in nature. The most frequent causes are traumatic injuries and infections in and about the joint. The ankylosis may be intra-articular or extra-articular. In intra-articular ankylosis the joint undergoes progressive destruction of the meniscus with flattening of the mandibular fossa, thickening of the head of the condyle and narrowing of the joint space. The ankylosis is basically fibrous, although ossification in the scar may result in a bony union. Extra-articular involvement is less frequently seen and produces an external fibrous or osseous encapsulation with minimal destruction of the joint itself.
Enumeratc thc ctiologic factors of TMJ ankylosis.

***Histopathologic Features:*** It is characterized by an excessive amount of dense, rather avascular fibrous connective tissue or new bone formation. Intra-articular ankylosis demonstrates irregular destruction of cartilage and bone with a sparse lymphocytic infiltration.

<u>**Inflammatory disturbances of TMJ**</u>

**Rheumatoid arthritis:** Rheumatoid arthritis is a chronic, presumably autoimmune disorder characterized by nonsuppurative inflammatory destruction of the joints. It affects women more frequently than men and may be a hypersensitivity reaction to bacterial toxins, specifically streptococci. Typically, the signs and symptoms become more severe over time and include swelling, stiffness, pain, joint deformity, and disability, with possible fibrous or bony fusion of opposing articular surfaces leading to ankylosis.

***Radiographic Features:*** Involved TMJs demonstrate a flattened condylar head with irregular surface features, an irregular temporal fossa surface, perhaps with remodelling of the fossa itself, and anterior displacement of the condyle.

***Histopathologic Features:*** The disease is characterized by the in growth of granulation tissue to cover the articular surfaces, the invasion of cartilage and its replacement by granulation tissue, and the ultimate destruction of the articular cartilage. When the TMJ is severely involved, the meniscus is typically perforated or replaced completely by fibrous scar.

**Osteoarthritis:** Osteoarthritis is a common degenerative and destructive alteration of the joints that was considered to be the result of simple wear and tear on aging anatomic structures. It is now known to have a strong inflammatory component as well, especially in small joints, such as the TMJ, where there appears to be little association with the aging process.

***Radiographic Appearance:*** Joints affected by osteoarthritis demonstrate a narrowing or obliteration of joint space, surface irregularities and protuberances (exostoses, osteophytes), flattening of the articular surface, osteosclerosis and osteolysis of bone beneath the cartilage.

***Histopathologic Features:*** The articulating surface of a joint affected by osteoarthritis has a diminished number of chondrocytes, is roughened, and contains variable numbers of vertical clefts; in older cases the clefts extend to the underlying bone. The cartilage cells often exhibit degeneration, and there may be complete destruction of cartilage in localized areas.

**Myofascial pain dysfunction syndrome**

Pain and dysfunction of the TMJ are common and have been proposed to result from a wide variety of etiologic factors, both traumatic and nontraumatic. The syndrome of signs and symptoms (pain, altered function, joint noises) is termed temporomandibular joint dysfunction (TMD) or myofascial pain dysfunction syndrome (MPD). Most patients complain of pain, which is usually localized to the preauricular area but may radiate to the temporal, frontal, or occipital areas. The pain may be a headache, a ringing in the ears (tinnitus), an earache (otalgia) or a toothache. The pain may be associated more with the surrounding musculature and soft tissue than with the TMJ itself. It is believed that the principal factor responsible for the manifestations of this syndrome is masticatory

muscle spasm. This muscle spasm can be initiated as a result of muscular overextension, muscular overcontraction or muscle fatigue. There are four positive signs and symptoms of this syndrome:

1. Pain
2. Muscle tenderness
3. A clicking or popping noise in the TMJ, and
4. Limitation of jaw motion sometimes with deviation.

There are two negative characteristics as well:

1. An absence of clinical, roentgenographic or biochemical evidence of organic changes in the joint itself, and
2. Lack of tenderness in the joint when it is palpated through the external auditory meatus. This disease is thought to have a psychologic or psychogenic component.

**Exercise Sixteen**

# DISEASES OF THE BLOOD

**Diseases involving the red blood cells**

**Anemia:** Define anemia. What are the types of anemia?

Enumerate the different laboratory investigations that are done to detect the cause of anemia.

**Pernicious anemia:** It is a common chronic disease presumably due to absence of "intrinsic factor" in the gastric juice of such patients as a result of which they are unable to absorb dietary vitamin $B_{12}$. The disease is characterized by generalized weakness, a sore and painful tongue, and numbness or tingling of the extremities.

Describe the oral manifestations of pernicious anemia.

**Peripheral blood smear:**

**Aplastic anemia:** Aplastic anemia is a rare, life-threating hematologic disorder that is characterized by failure of the haematopoietic precursor cell in the bone marrow to produce adequate numbers of all types of blood cells. The clinical manifestations of the disease vary according to the type of cell chiefly affected.

Describe the clinical features and oral manifestations of aplastic anemia.

**Thalassemia:** Thalassemia represents a group of disorders of hemoglobin synthesis that are characterized by reduced synthesis of either the alpha-globin or beta-globin chains of the hemoglobin molecule. The abnormal erythrocytes are destroyed by the spleen (hemolytic) and the patient suffers from hypo chromic, microcytic anemia.

Describe the clinical and radiographic features of thalassemia.

**Sickle cell anemia:** It is one of the more severe genetic disorders of hemoglobin synthesis (hemoglobinopathies). Normal adult hemoglobin (HbA) is genetically altered to produce sickle hemoglobin (HbS) by the substitution of valine for glutamine at the sixth position of the β-globin chain.

Describe the clinical features of sickle cell anemia.

**Blood smear:** Typical sickle shaped red blood cells are commonly seen.

## Diseases involving the white blood cells

**Leukopenia:** It is an abnormal reduction in the number of white blood cells in the peripheral blood stream. This decrease involves predominantly the granulocytes and the number of circulating neutrophils goes below $1500/mm^3$ in an adult.

Enumerate the causes of neutropenia.

**Agranulocytosis:** Agranulocytosis is a condition in which the cells of the granulocyte series, mainly the neutrophils, are absent. Agranulocytosis may occur as a result of decreased production or increased destruction or use of these cells. Primary agranulocytosis is that form of the disease in which the etiology is unknown while in secondary agranulocytosis the etiology is recognized.

Name the drugs, which have been reported to produce agranulocytosis.

**Oral manifestations:** Oral lesions are common and include necrotizing, deep punched out ulcerations of the buccal mucosa, tongue and palate.

***Histopathologic Features:*** The microscopic appearance of oral ulcerations in agranulocytosis shows abundant bacterial organisms, both on the surface and within the tissue. The host inflammatory response is sparse with few granulocytes seen in the ulcer bed.

**Leukemia:** Leukemia is a disease characterized by the progressive overproduction of white blood cells, which usually appear in the circulating blood in an immature form. Leukemias are broadly classified as acute or chronic (according to the clinical course) and myeloid or lymphocytic/lymphoblastic (according to the histogenetic origin). Myeloid leukemias can differentiate along several different pathways producing malignant cells that usually show features of granulocytes or monocytes, and less frequently, erythrocytes or megakaryocytes. Many of the clinical signs and symptoms of leukemia are related to the marked reduction in the numbers of normal white and red blood cells, a phenomenon that results from the crowding out of the normal hematopoietic stem cells by the malignant proliferation. Megakaryocytes are also crowded out of the marrow resulting in thrombocytopenia.

Describe the oral manifestations of leukemia.

***Histopathologic Features:*** Microscopic examination of leukemia-affected tissue shows diffuse infiltration and destruction of the normal host tissue by sheets of poorly differentiated cells with either myelomonocytic characteristics or lymphoid features.

**Diseases involving the blood platelets**

**Purpura:** Purpura is defined as a purplish discoloration of the skin and mucous membranes due to the spontaneous extravasation of blood and, in itself, is a symptom rather than a disease entity. If the platelets are defective or deficient purpura may result. It may be classified as:

1. Nonthrombocytopenic purpura
2. Thrombocytopenic purpura
   a. Primary or "essential" purpura
   b. Secondary or symptomatic purpura.

What are the oral manifestations and laboratory findings of thrombocytopenic purpura?

**Diseases involving specific blood factors**

**Haemophilia:** Deficiency of which factor causes haemophilia? Write the clinical features and laboratory findings of haemophilia.

**von Willebrand's disease (Pseudohemophilia):** von Willebrand's disease is characterized by the tendency to excessive bleeding in patients who have a normal platelet count, normal clotting time, normal serum fibrinogen and normal prothrombin time. Only the bleeding time is prolonged. Whereas classic hemophilia is caused by a deficiency of only one of the components of factor VIII, classic von Willebrand's disease is caused by decreases in all three functional components of factor VIII.

Write the clinical features and laboratory findings of von Willebrand's disease.

# DISEASES OF THE PERIODONTIUM

Periodontal diseases are classified into two general groups on the basis of the pathologic processes present:

1. Inflammation (gingivitis and periodontitis), and
2. Dystrophy (gingivosis and periodontosis, now usually termed "juvenile periodontitis"). The etiology of the inflammatory periodontal diseases is varied, but is usually divided into local factors and/or systemic factors, which provoke or aggravate the inflammatory reaction. Dystrophic or regressive changes of the periodontium are caused by degenerative, circulatory or mechanical influences, or by other abnormalities, which result in pathologic changes in the periodontium.

**Pellicle:** The acquired pellicle is a thin deposit, which may form shortly after eruption on the exposed surfaces of teeth.

Name and give causes for the different types of extrinsic stains on the teeth.

**Calculus:** Calculus is attached dental plaque, which has undergone mineralization. They are hard stone-like concretions formed on teeth or prosthetic appliances in the oral cavity.

What is the composition of calculus?

**Gingivitis:** Gingivitis is the inflammation of marginal and attached gingiva surrounding the teeth.
Enumerate the local and systemic etiologic factors of gingivitis.

***Histopathologic Features:*** The connective tissue of the gingiva is infiltrated by varying numbers of lymphocytes, monocytes and plasma cells in chronic gingivitis. Polymorphonuclear leucocytes are occasionally noted particularly beneath the crevicular epithelium. The capillaries are usually engorged and sometimes increased in number. Edema of the connective tissue may be prominent.

**Acute necrotizing ulcerative gingivitis (ANUG):** Necrotizing ulcerative gingivitis has a distinctive pattern of gingival pathologic changes that have been recognized for hundreds of years. Fusobacterium nucleatum and Borrelia vincenti have been identified as the causative organisms. The infection frequently occurs in the presence of psychologic stress. Other related factors are immunosuppression, smoking, local trauma, poor nutritional status, poor oral hygiene, inadequate sleep and recent illness. The interdental papillae are highly inflamed, edematous, and hemorrhagic. Typically the affected papillae are blunted and demonstrate areas of "punched-out", craterlike necrosis that are covered with a gray pseudomembrane.

***Histopathologic Features:*** Features of ANUG are not specific. Affected gingival papillae show surface ulceration that is covered by a thickened fibrinopurulent membrane. The underlying lamina propria demonstrates an intense acute or mixed inflammatory infiltrate and extensive hyperemia.

**Gingival hyperplasia:** Gingival hyperplasia may be: (1) Inflammatory gingival hyperplasia, (2) Noninflammatory or fibrous gingival hyperplasia, and (3) Combination of inflammatory and fibrous hyperplasias.

**Inflammatory gingival hyperplasia:** This usually results from prolonged chronic inflammation of the gingival tissues. The nature of the chronic irritation causing the hyperplasia may be variable but the histologic picture is usually nonspecific, showing merely inflammation of the gingiva. The inflammatory hyperplasia has been associated with vitamin C deficiency, leukemia, endocrine imbalance and Crohn's disease.

**Fibrous gingival hyperplasia:** The gingiva shows no tendency to bleed and surface is well stippled and of normal colour. Microscopically the enlargement is primarily due to an increase in the bulk of mature fibrous connective tissue. The etiologic factor may be known or idiopathic.

Name the drugs causing fibrous hyperplasia of gingiva.

**Periodontitis:** Periodontitis refers to an inflammation of the gingival tissues in association with some loss of both the attachment of the periodontal ligament and bony support. Apical migration of the crevicular epithelium along the root surface results in the formation of periodontal pockets. Loosening and eventual loss of teeth may take place. Periodontitis may be classified as:

1. Chronic periodontitis
2. Aggressive periodontitis
3. Periodontitis as a manifestation of systemic disease
4. Necrotizing periodontal diseases
5. Abscesses of the periodontium
6. Periodontitis associated with endodontic lesions.

***Histopathologic Features:*** Gingivitis is present with hyperplasia of crevicular epithelium lining the pocket and intense acute inflammatory cell infiltration. The adjacent connective tissue shows an increased vascularity and inflammatory cellular infiltration of mixed type. Frequently large colonies of microorganisms are noted.

**Juvenile periodontitis:** It is defined by Baer as "a disease of the periodontium which can occur in an otherwise healthy adolescent, which is characterized by a rapid loss of alveolar bone about more than one tooth of the permanent dentition. The amount of destruction manifested is not commensurate with the amount of local irritants present."

Presently the term "Aggressive periodontitis" has replaced the older term "juvenile periodontitis". Suspected pathogens found in aggressive periodontitis are A. actinomycetemcomitans, P. intermedia, P. gingivalis and some less common organisms.

**Localized aggressive periodontitis:** It begins around the ages of 11 to 13 years and has a strong familial tendency with attachment loss localized to the first molars and incisors.

**Generalized aggressive periodontitis:** This condition may not represent a distinct disease entity but may be a collection of young adults with advanced periodontal disease. There is generalized loss of attachment that must affect at least three teeth other than the first molars and incisors.

***Histopathologic Features:*** Microscopically the picture is similar to chronic periodontitis. Possibility of other systemic disease to be ruled out.

**Exercise Eighteen**

# DISEASES OF THE SKIN

**Hereditary ectodermal dysplasia:** It is a specific syndrome characterized by a congenital dysplasia of one or more ectodermal structures and their accessory appendages, manifested primarily by hypohidrosis, hypotrichosis and hypodontia.

***Histopathologic Features:*** Histopathologic examination of the skin from a patient with ectodermal dysplasia shows a decreased number of sweat glands and hair follicles. The adnexal structures that are present are hypoplastic and malformed.

Describe the oral manifestations of hereditary ectodermal dysplasia.

**White sponge nevus:** It is a relatively rare genetically determined skin disorder characterized by a defect in the normal keratinization of the oral mucosa. Symmetric, thickened, white, corrugated or velvety, diffuse plaques affect the buccal mucosa bilaterally in most cases.

***Histopathologic Features:*** Prominent hyperparakeratosis and marked acanthosis with clearing of the cytoplasm of the spinous layer cells are common features but not pathognomonic of white sponge nevus. Sometimes, an eosinophilic condensation is noted in the perinuclear region of the cells in the superficial layers of the epithelium, which is unique to this lesion.

**Lichen planus:** Lichen planus is a relatively common, chronic dermatologic disease that often affects the oral mucosa. Though the etiology of lichen planus is not known but stress and anxiety have been closely associated with this condition. Current evidence indicates that this is an immunologically mediated mucocutaneous disorder. The skin papules reveal a fine, lacelike network of white lines (Wickham's striae) while the oral lesions may be of either reticular or erosive forms.

***Histopathologic Features:*** The characteristic microscopic features of lichen planus are varying degrees of ortho or parakeratosis with pointed or "saw toothed" shape of rete pegs. Destruction of the basal cell layer of the epithelium accompanied by an intense, bandlike infiltrate of predominantly T lymphocytes in the subepithelial region of connective tissue. Civatte bodies or degenerating keratinocytes may be seen in the epithelium and connective tissue interface.

**Psoriasis:** It is a common chronic skin disease, which rarely manifests in the oral mucosa. Psoriasis is characterized by an increased proliferative activity of the cutaneous keratinocytes. Skin lesions are characterized by the occurrence of small dry papules covered by a delicate silvery scale which when removed disclose one or more tiny bleeding points. This is a characteristic feature of the disease termed Auspitz's sign.

***Histopathologic Features:*** Microscopically, psoriasis is characterized by marked keratin production and elongated rete ridges. The connective tissue papillae containing dilated capillaries approach close to the epithelial surface with the presence of a perivascular chronic inflammatory cell infiltrate. Intraepithelial microabscesses (Munro abscess) is a common finding.

**Erythema multiforme:** Erythema multiforme is a vesiculobullous mucocutaneous condition of uncertain etiopathogenesis. Herpes simplex infection may precede the condition by two to three weeks. Erythematous skin lesions appear as concentric circular rings resembling a target or bull's eye (target lesions). The oral lesions appear as erythematous patches, which evolve into shallow erosions and ulcerations.

**Stevens-Johnson syndrome:** A more severe form of the disease is usually triggered by a drug rather than infection. Stevens-Johnson syndrome is a very severe bullous form of erythema multiforme with widespread involvement of skin, oral cavity, eyes and genitalia.

***Histopathologic Features:*** The microscopic appearance is not pathognomonic. Subepithelial or intraepithelial vesiculation may be seen in association with necrotic basal keratinocytes with frequent absence of the basement membrane. A mixed inflammatory infiltrate is present with dilatation of superficial capillaries in the connective tissue.

**Pemphigus:** Pemphigus is an autoimmune disorder manifested by vesiculobullous lesions that develop in cycles. The various types of pemphigus are: Pemphigus vulgaris, Pemphigus vegetans, Pemphigus foliaceous and Pemphigus erythematosus. Only the vulgaris and vegetans types affect the oral mucosa. The oral lesions are often the first sign of the disease. Autoantibodies are produced against the epidermal desmosomes resulting in splitting of the epithelium with blister formation.

Describe the clinical features of pemphigus vulgaris.

***Histopathologic Features:*** Pemphigus is characterized microscopically by intraepithelial vesicle or bulla formation producing suprabasilar split. The cells of the spinous layer show acantholysis with the loose cells assuming a rounded shape called Tzanck cells which are identified in an Exfoliative cytologic preparation.

**Cicatricial pemphigoid (Benign mucous membrane pemphigoid):** It is suggested that cicatricial pemphigoid represents a group of chronic, blistering, mucocutaneous autoimmune diseases in which tissue-bound autoantibodies are directed against one or more components of the basement membrane. The vesiculobullous lesions occur on the skin, oral mucosa and conjunctiva.

***Histopathologic Features:*** The vesicles and bullae are subepidermal rather than suprabasilar and there is no acantholysis. The basement membrane structure appears to detach with the epithelium from the underlying connective tissue. A mild chronic inflammatory cell infiltrate is present in the superficial submucosa.

**Bullous pemphigoid:** Bullous pemphigoid is the most common of the autoimmune blistering conditions. It is characterized by the production of autoantibodies directed against components of the basement membrane. It has many features common with cicatricial pemphigoid with a significant difference being in the clinical course of the disease. The clinical course in patients with bullous pemphigoid is usually limited whereas the course in patients with cicatricial pemphigoid is usually protracted and progressive.

***Histopathologic Features:*** The vesicles and bullae in this disease are subepidermal and nonspecific with no evidence of acantholytic epithelial cells. The presence of eosinophils within the bulla itself is a characteristic feature with moderate degree of mixed inflammatory infiltrate in the lesional area.

**Epidermolysis bullosa:** Epidermolysis bullosae is an uncommon group of mucocutaneous disease in which bullae or vesicles appear spontaneously or after minor trauma. There is a specific defect in the attachment mechanisms of the epithelial cells, either to each other or to underlying connective tissue. Depending upon the defective mechanism of cellular cohesion, there are three broad categories: Simplex, Junctional and Dystrophic.

***Histopathologic Features:*** The simplex form shows intraepithelial clefting by light microscopy while junctional and dystrophic forms show subepithelial clefting.

**Lupus erythematosus:** Lupus erythematosus is a "collagen vascular" or "connective tissue" disease, which is immunologically mediated. It exists in two basic forms namely systemic lupus erythematosus and discoid lupus erythematosus.

**Systemic lupus erythematosus:** Women are affected nearly 10 times more frequently than men. There is a characteristic butterfly rash across the bridge of the nose. Cutaneous lesions may present itching or burning sensation with areas of hyperpigmentation the severity of which is intensified with exposure to sunlight. The generalized manifestations are related to involvement of various organs including the kidney and heart.

**Discoid lupus erythematosus:** Oral mucous membrane, skin of the face, neck and back are more commonly involved. The cutaneous lesions are elevated red macules frequently covered by gray or yellow adherent scales the forceful removal of which reveals numerous "carpet tack" extensions which had dipped into enlarged pilosebaceous canals. Butterfly rash may be evident across the bridge of the nose in the discoid form as well.

***Histopathologic Features:*** The oral lesions demonstrate hyperkeratosis, alternating atrophy and thickening of the spinous cell layer, degeneration of the basal cell layer, and subepithelial lymphocytic infiltration. These features are similar to lichen planus and differentiation between the two conditions are done by the presence of PAS-positive material in the basement membrane zone in lupus erythematosus along with subepithelial oedema and a more diffuse and deeper inflammatory infiltrate.

What are the laboratory findings in lupus erythematosus?

**Systemic sclerosis:** Systemic sclerosis is a condition that probably has an immunologically mediated pathogenesis. Raynaud's phenomenon is often one of the first signs of progressive systemic sclerosis where the hands and face are involved, but the feet are seldom affected. Dense collagen is deposited in the body tissues in excessive amounts resulting in vasoconstriction. The skin develops a diffuse hard texture with a smooth surface resulting in a mask-like facies. Microstomia often develops as a result of collagen deposition in the perioral tissues.

***Radiographic Features:*** Diffuse widening of the periodontal ligament space is often present throughout the dentition.

***Histopathologic Features:*** The condition is characterized microscopically by diffuse deposition of dense collagen within and around normal structures causing loss of normal tissue function.

Exercise Ninteen

# DISEASES OF NERVES

**Trigeminal neuralgia:** It is a disease involving the fifth cranial nerve supplying the teeth, jaws, face and associated structures.

Describe the clinical features of trigeminal neuralgia. What are trigger zones?

**Auriculotemporal syndrome:** Frey's syndrome is an unusual phenomenon, which arises as a result of damage to the auriculotemporal nerve and subsequent reinnervation of sweat glands by parasympathetic salivary fibres. The patient typically exhibits flushing and sweating of the involved side of the face, mainly in the temporal region, during eating.

What is the etiology of this condition?

**Bell's palsy:** This condition is caused by the paralysis of seventh cranial nerve supplying the muscles of the face. Though the cause of this condition remains unknown but cases have been reported where Bell's palsy was precipitated after exposure to cold.
Describe the clinical features of Bell's palsy.

**Glossopharyngeal neuralgia:** Pain similar to that of trigeminal neuralgia may arise from the disturbance of ninth cranial nerve. The patient usually has a "trigger zone" in the posterior oropharynx or tonsillar fossa. The etiology of glossopharyngeal neuralgia is unknown.

**Exercise Twenty**

# DISEASES OF THE MUSCLES

**Myasthenias:** Myasthenia is an abnormal weakness and fatigue in muscle following activity. These constitute a group of diseases in which there is a basic disorder of muscle excitability and contractility and include:

1. Myasthenia gravis
2. Familial periodic paralysis
3. Aldosteronism.

Describe the clinical features of myasthenia gravis.

Exercise Twenty One

# FORENSIC ODONTOLOGY

**Forensic Odontology** has been defined by the Federation Dentaire Internationale (FDI) as 'that branch of dentistry which, in the interest of justice, deals with the proper handling and examination of dental evidence, and with the proper evaluation and presentation of dental findings.' Forensic odontologists deal with:

1. Identification of unknown human remains through ante mortem and post mortem dental records
2. Victim identification at the scene of crime
3. Determination of ethnicity at archeological sites
4. Sex assessment of skeletal remains
5. Age estimation
6. Bite mark analysis
7. Expert witness in presenting evidence in court of law.

**Personal Identification**

Identification helps in establishing a person's individuality.

What is personal identification and what are the traditional methods of identification?

**Dental Identification**

1. ***Comparative dental identification:*** Postmortem dental identification includes:
    (a) Oral autopsy
    (b) Obtaining dental records
    (c) Comparing ante- and post-mortem dental data
    (d) Writing a report and drawing conclusion

A range of conclusions can be drawn namely-

Positive Identification:

Probable Identification:

Possible Identification:

Insufficient Information:

Excludes Identification:

**Ameloglyphics**

The study of tooth prints formed by the enamel rod ends at the surface of tooth crown is known as Ameloglyphics.

**Dental DNA in Identification**

DNA can be successfully extracted from the pulp of teeth recovered from mutilated, burned or decomposed bodies. PCR (polymerase chain reaction) is the technique employed in amplifying minute quantities or even highly degraded DNA. In absence of decedent's antemortem sample, DNA can be compared to that of parents or siblings to achieve confirmative identification.

What are the methods of dental DNA extraction?

**Study of palatal rugae pattern**

Identification of edentulous patients can be done by Rugoscopy or the study of palatal rugae pattern. Palatal rugae are ridges on the anterior part of the palatal mucosa on each side of the mid-palatine raphae, behind the incisive papilla. Rugae pattern are considered unique to an individual. They seldom change shape with age and reappear after trauma or surgical procedures. Lysell's classification of rugae pattern:

- Primary rugae (>5mm)
- Secondary rugae (3-5mm)
- Fragmentary rugae (2<3mm)

  (Rugae <2mm is not considered)

***Exercise:*** Trace the rugae pattern in any given cast and analyse the pattern obtained.

**Dental Profiling**

According to Pretty and Sweet Dental profiling includes extracting a triad of information namely, decedent's ethnic origin, sex and age and the information obtained from this process enables a more focused search for antemortem records.

What are the means of determining ethnic origin from teeth?

***Sex determination:*** Sex can be determined by assessing the data from morphology of skull and mandible, tooth measurements and DNA analysis from teeth.

***Dental age estimation:*** Dental age estimation makes use of morphologic, radiographic, histological, and biochemical methods to analyse age changes in teeth.

Write about Schour and Massler's method of dental age estimation.

What is Demirjian's method of age estimation?

What are the methods of age estimation in adults?

Name some biochemical indicators of age.

## Crime Investigation

Forensic odontologists play a vital role in crime investigation. Crime investigation includes the investigation of bite marks, child abuse, and lip prints.

***Bite marks:*** MacDonald defined bite marks as, "a mark caused by the teeth either alone or in combination with other mouth parts."

What are the different classification systems of bite marks?

***Exercise:*** Analyse the bite mark obtained on wax sheet/ food stuff. Draw the bite mark imprint.

***Lip prints:*** Study of lip prints is known as, 'cheiloscopy'. Lip prints are produced by the grooves on the lips and are heritable and individualistic. They constitute material evidence left at a crime scene similar to fingerprints.

***Classification:*** According to Tsuchihashi the pattern of grooves are of six types:

Type I- Vertical grooves that run across the entire lip

Type I'- Similar to type I but do not cover the entire lip

Type II- Branched grooves

Type III- Intersected grooves

Type IV- Reticular grooves

Type V- Grooves that cannot be morphologically differentiated

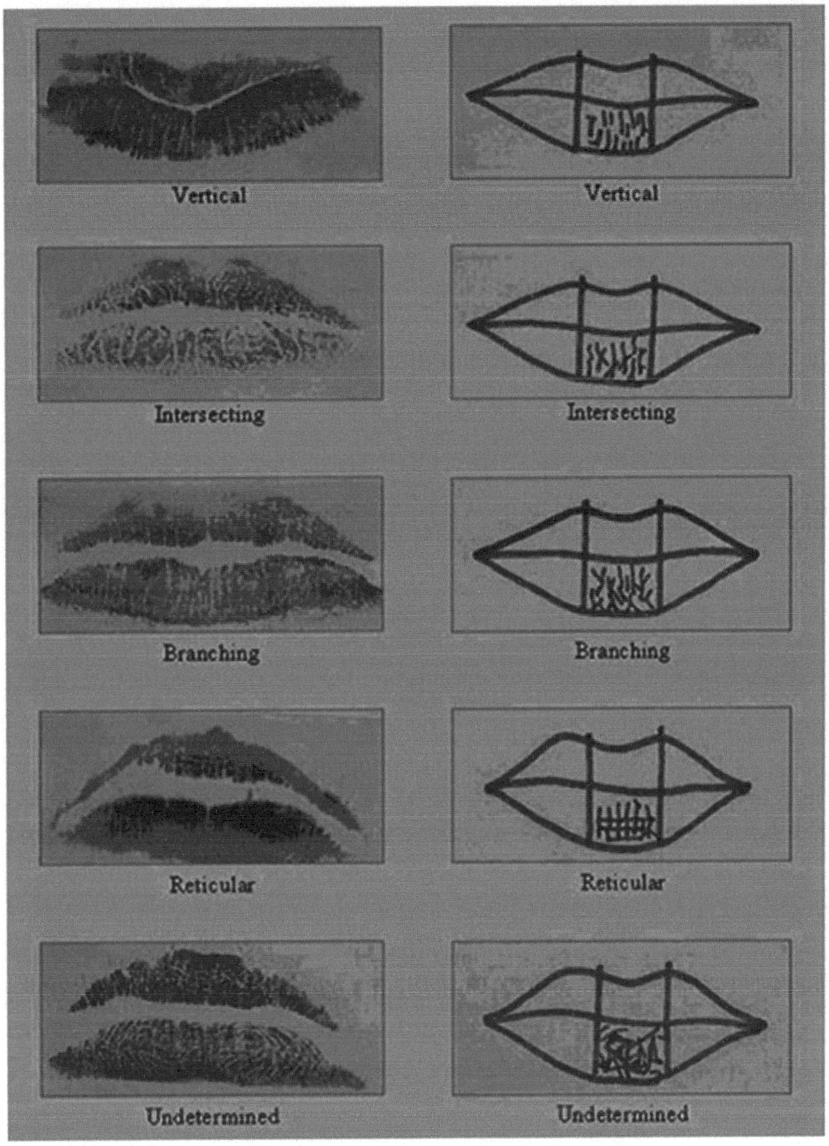


**Fig. Showing types of lip prints**

***Exercise:*** Take a lip print and classify the groove pattern.

As experts, dentists may need to testify in cases involving malpractice, dental fraud, accidents and injuries, in addition to post-mortem identification, age estimation and bite mark investigation. An additional knowledge and experience is essential for qualifying as a forensic expert, if not a recognized qualification or board certification.